Essential Guide to Behçet's Disease

Written and compiled by
Joanne Zeis

Dedicated to:
Mike, Ben and Sarah, always.
Sue, Anne-Marie and Beth;
my BD friends;
and the women of Silver Scissors.

**With grateful acknowledgement to those who reviewed
the manuscript and provided valuable suggestions:**
C. Stephen Foster, M.D., F.A.C.S.; Kenneth T. Calamia, M.D.;
Susan N. Legacy, M.D.; Bettina Bailey, M.S.W., L.I.C.S.W.;
Lisa Jensen, M.P.H.; Susan Sharrow, R.N.

In memory of:
Lynn Acquaviva-Sisk
Diane Romano, and
LuAnne Klemme, M.D.
who gave so much, and left too soon.

*Faith is being sure of what we hope for,
and certain of what we do not see. (Hebrews 11:1)*

Essential Guide to Behçet's Disease
Copyright 2003 by Joanne Zeis

Central Vision Press
PO Box 255
Uxbridge, MA 01569-0255
www.centralvisionpress.com

ISBN 0-9658403-3-6
Library of Congress Control No:
2002092326

Other books and resources by Joanne Zeis:
You Are Not Alone: 15 People with Behçet's
Basic Information on Behçet's Disease
Behçet's Disease: Medical Research Studies
www. behcetsdisease.com

FOREWORD

Behçet's disease is an unusual multisystem disease that is rare outside of Asia and the Mediterranean basin. Yet individuals in nearly all parts of the world have been reported with this chronic and relapsing disorder, which can produce enormous life-altering consequences to the individual with it. The disease is frustrating, to patient and physician alike. Because of its relative rarity in America, few physicians have had the opportunity to care for even a single patient with Behçet's disease, much less 10 or 20 or 100, over an extended period. Therefore, few physicians in America have the experience of diagnosing, let alone treating, patients with Behçet's disease. Additionally, the disorder may be found in many different forms and levels of severity: some never having eye involvement, some relatively mild, with primarily joint and oral mucosal involvement, and some producing truly cataclysmic life-threatening lesions of vital organs.

The ***Essential Guide to Behçet's Disease*** is a resource unlike any other to my knowledge. It is a treasury of information, primarily of established fact, gleaned from the medical literature. It also contains a small amount of non-medical material, including references on herbal and alternative treatment options. And finally it holds, in its appendices, concrete, valuable information on the details of how one applies for Social Security Disability benefits, as well as resources for contacting other organizations devoted to the support of patients with Behçet's disease.

This extraordinary reference guide will be of enormous value to every patient (and their family members) with Behçet's disease. Additionally, and without any negative connotations whatsoever, it may also be helpful to those physicians caring for a patient with Behçet's disease for the first time.

C. Stephen Foster, M.D., F.A.C.S.
Professor of Ophthalmology,
Harvard Medical School
Director, Immunology and Uveitis Service,
Massachusetts Eye and Ear Infirmary,
Boston, Massachusetts

i

This book is the culmination of over twenty years of personal experience and research on the art, and science, of living with Behçet's disease. While I am not medically trained, a lifelong interest in the medical field has made it possible for me to sift through piles of research reports over the years, in a quest for the most patient-oriented information available on BD - the type of information that I have used in the past to create other books and resources on Behçet's for patients, their friends, family members, and healthcare providers.

It is not my intention for the information in this book to replace any patient's relationship with his or her primary care physician. I continually encourage patients to discuss questions that they may have about symptoms or treatments with their health care provider(s). My strong personal interest in the field of Behçet's does not include a license to offer medical advice. As such, I have relied heavily in this book on research results published by medical experts in their areas of interest. Every effort has been made to accurately record these research results, but human nature dictates that occasional mistakes may slip through the cracks. Please contact me with any suggested corrections or revisions, so that text changes can be made before the printing of future editions.

I hope that your search for information on Behçet's disease is made easier with this book, and that you find a measure of comfort in the details.

Be well,

Joanne Zeis

TABLE OF CONTENTS

(continued on next page)

Table of contents

Essential Guide to Behçet's Disease

CHAPTER 1

Frequently-asked questions about Behçet's disease

How do you pronounce "Behçet's" ?
The most popular pronunciations are Beh SHETS, Beh SHAY, and Beh
SETS. Ironically, the correct Turkish pronunciation - Beh **CHETS** - is
rarely used by English-speaking physicians or patients. Some researchers are now referring to the illness as Beh CHET disease (without the **s**).[151]

What is Behçet's?
Behçet's disease (BD) is a rare and chronic multisystem disorder that
causes the inflammation of blood vessels anywhere in the body. This
inflammation is known as vasculitis. For the most part, the location of
the inflammation(s) is what dictates a patient's symptoms. The most
common symptoms include aphthous ulcers of the mouth and genitals,
along with uveitis (a form of eye inflammation). This grouping, known
as the "triple-symptom complex," was widely published in 1937 as a
unique disease by the Turkish dermatologist, Hulusi Behçet, although
other physicians — including Bluthe and Adamantiades, a Greek
ophthalmologist— wrote of patients with these combined health issues
prior to 1937.[150] Adamantiades, in particular, published details in the
1931 French ophthalmic literature of a case with Behçet's-like features.
He suggested that the symptoms were part of a distinct disease process,
but his paper was not as well-distributed as the later one by Behcet.
Hence, for all but a few stalwart Adamantiades supporters, the disease
carries only Behçet's name.[220] We now know that BD encompasses a
much wider range of medical problems beyond the originally-described
three symptoms.

　　　Behçet's disease typically starts when patients are in their 20s
and 30s, but it has been seen in all ages from infants to the elderly.
Some families may have more than one blood relative who displays
partial or full BD symptoms, although this situation is supposedly
uncommon. More information on familial connections can be found in
the chapter on *Behçet's in Families*.

　　　BD is a long-term, unpredictable, and cyclical disease that
comes and goes in "flares" of varying instensities. There may be symptom-free periods of weeks or months that are interrupted by flares
lasting a few days, weeks, or months. In this cyclical sense, Behçet's is

1

much like multiple sclerosis or lupus. Some people can be hospitalized at times with the more serious complications of BD, but there are also occasional reports of people who go into permanent remission. As you can see, it's all very uncertain.

However, most Behçet's patients deal with some level of symptoms for their entire lives. At the present time, there is no way to predict which patients will move on to more serious problems, which ones will remain stable, and which ones might go into remission.

Individual cases of Behçet's are sometimes categorized by the most prominent disease feature that the patient is experiencing. For example, a "neuro-Behçet" patient is primarily dealing with complications of the central nervous system.

How many people have Behçet's?

The reported incidence of Behçet's disease has stayed fairly consistent over the years:

(Incidence figures in first three rows from footnote 1; case calculations based on population statistics from footnote 2.

Japan	1/10,000 people =	approximately 13,000	cases
Middle East	1/10,000 =	approximately 27,000	cases
USA	0.5/10,000 =	approximately 14,000	cases
UK	approximately 2000 cases [73]		

Is Behçet's contagious?

No. It's not possible to "catch" Behçet's from touching, being near, or sharing food with someone who has BD. Once herpes or other sexually transmitted diseases have been ruled out as a possible cause of genital lesions, sexual intimacy is also safe - although intercourse may be painful for the patient if genital ulcers are present.

My doctor says only people from the Middle East or Japan can have Behçet's.

Behçet's disease tends to strike people with "Silk Road" bloodlines more frequently than it affects people of other ancestries. Silk Road countries include those in the Mediterranean basin, Middle East, and Far East. However, cases of Behçet's disease (or syndrome) have been found worldwide, regardless of patients' backgrounds. Therefore, a Behçet's diagnosis should not be ruled out in anyone who displays the primary symptoms outlined in the International Criteria for Behçet's Disease (described later) - even if the patient doesn't have a traditional Silk Road heritage.

Questions occasionally arise about the association between Behçet's disease and the Melungeon people of the Appalachians in the southeastern US. According to N. Brent Kennedy (1997), "Melungeons are a people of apparent Mediterranean descent who may have settled in the Appalachian wilderness as early as, or possibly earlier than, 1567."[245] There was almost certainly intermarriage over the years between native American tribal members and Melungeon descendants. Specific native American tribes mentioned by Kennedy include the Powhatans, Pamunkeys, Creeks, Catawbas, Yuchis, and Cherokees. Several Mediterranean diseases are known to afflict Melungeons, including Familial Mediterranean Fever, thalassemia, and Behçet's disease. More information on the Melungeon people can be found at the Melungeon Health Education and Support web site at www.melungeonhealth.org.

Is Behçet's disease the same as Behçet's syndrome?
Physicians and patients often use the terms interchangeably, although this practice has caused some dispute. At the Ninth International Conference on Behçet's Disease (Korea, 2000), Lee noted that Behçet's is more often termed a "disease" than a "syndrome" in papers published on the topic. According to Lee's study group, 2,228 papers related to Behçet's have been published in the past sixty years; the term "disease" was used in 71% of the papers, while "syndrome" was used in the remaining 29%. The study group recommended the adoption of a unified terminology from this point forward, and that Behçet's be declared a disease rather than a syndrome.[104]

Lee's group also gathered opinions on this topic from 22 board members of the International Study Group for Behçet's Disease. While almost all members agreed on the "disease" terminology, one holdout stated that only people of Mediterranean, Middle Eastern or Far Eastern heritage can have a true case of Behçet's *disease*; and that people from other parts of the world have Behçet's *syndrome*-a group of symptoms similar to those found in Behçet's disease, but with a different etiology (cause).

Behçet's disease is also known by several other names: Triple-symptom complex, Adamantiades-Behçet disease,[5] Silk Road disease, and Morbus Behçet (the Latin translation of "Behçet's disease"), among others.

Who gets Behçet's more frequently, men or women?
 In the Silk Road countries, Behçet's disease has traditionally been more common in men than in women. For example, studies in Israel and Japan found the male-to-female ratio to be 4.9:1, and 1.7:1, respectively. In a 1975 worldwide review of 683 Behçet's patients, men outnumbered women at a rate of 2.3:1. However, studies in the UK and US in the 1970s showed an opposite trend, with female cases outnumbering male cases. The male-to-female ratios in these studies were 0.6:1 (UK) and 0.4:1 (US)[4]

A current study by Haskard (2001) reports a shift towards a more equal male/female gender distribution in the UK - a finding that he says coincides with results also found in European and Turkish studies.[73] Some other recent studies still reaffirm the old trends: in Iraq (Sharquie et al, 2000), the male:female ratio is 2.9:1;[74] and in Jordan (Madanat, 2000), the male:female ratio is 3:1.[75]

3

Is Behçet's disease hereditary?

Behçet's disease appears to have a genetic component but is not passed to future generations in the same way as, for example, a disease like hemophilia or sickle cell anemia. Researchers believe that some people have a genetic predisposition to developing Behçet's — but that an environmental element, an unknown virus, or perhaps a bacterial infection is needed to actually trigger the disease in these predisposed people.

If it's not strictly hereditary, then what causes Behçet's disease?

To date, no one has successfully identified the "trigger" that creates a case of Behçet's in someone with a genetic predisposition for BD. In 1989, Cooper et al performed a research study asking "Is Behçet's disease triggered by childhood infection?" In their comparison of 30 BD patients with 60 age- and sex-matched healthy subjects, "an increased risk of Behçet's disease was associated with tonsillectomy, a history of cold sores, large sibship size [many siblings], late birth order, travel to countries with high incidence of the disease, and first sexual intercourse before 16 years of age. These findings are consistent with a triggering of the disease by infection during childhood or adolescence in an immunogenetically predisposed host."[182]

Researchers have performed many studies while trying to identify the possible trigger that might lead to Behçet's in genetically predisposed people. Streptococcus sanguis has been suggested in several studies,[183] as well as the herpes simplex virus.[184] Streptococcus sanguis should not be confused with bacterial strep throat from a contagious source, however, as S. sanguis bacteria are part of the normal human oral microflora.[221] More recent research has looked at the possible involvement of heat shock proteins (HSP), which are created by living cells as a protective response to "heat, anoxia [lack of oxygen], toxic metabolites and other causes of stress which may result from infection."(Lehner, 2001)[185] In 2001, Ergun et al found statistically significant levels of HSP 60/65 in the biopsied skin lesions of patients with active cases of Behçet's disease, and they recommend further study on the matter.[186]

Why do you keep putting the letters "et al" after people's names? It's really annoying.

"Et al" is used to show that there were other people involved in creating and carrying out a particular research study. In many cases, it would take up too much space to list all of the researchers, so only the first one or two names on the published paper appear here in the text.

What types of symptoms show up most frequently in Behçet's patients?

Kaklamani and Kaklamanis (2001) compiled the results of six specific research studies performed on a total of 8,039 BD patients between 1970 and 2001.[59]

Symptom	Prevalence
Oral ulcers	96-100% of cases
Genital ulcers	64-82%
Skin lesions	74-87%
Ocular lesions	47-73%
Arthritis	40-64%
CNS involvement	3-20%
Vasculitis	6-38%
GI involvement	4-20% *
Epididymo-orchitis	6-22% **
Positive pathergy test	37-62% ***

CNS=central nervous system; GI=gastrointestinal
*One study of 601 patients (7% of total 8039 patients reviewed) did not report on GI involvement
**Two studies totaling 1097 patients (14% of total 8039 patients reviewed) did not report on epididymoorchitis
***One study of 496 patients (6% of total 8039 patients reviewed) did not report on pathergy test results

Why do the statistics look like that? For example, why does the list say that "3-20%" of patients have CNS (central nervous system) involvement?

The statistics in this example show a *range* of the results from six research studies that were performed in different countries. In this case, the fewest number of patients with CNS symptoms in any of the reviewed studies was 3%. The greatest number of patients with CNS symptoms in any of the studies was 20%. So — if there were 100 patients in each of these studies, then three patients had CNS symptoms in the first study, and twenty patients had CNS problems in the last study. *[JZ: Kocer et al (1999) made mention of a 4-49% range of CNS involvement,[137] showing that results can vary widely between research studies. In addition, research results can be influenced by the location of the original study and the heritage of the enrolled patients, as some symptoms can be seen more commonly in some parts of the world than in others.][21]*

Is there any test that can definitely diagnose a case of Behçet's?

No. Behçet's is considered a disease of "exclusion" - doctors try to eliminate the other diseases that you might have (lupus, MS and Crohn's are big contenders) and then see if your symptoms still fall in line with the standard health problems found in Behcet's. There are some tests that might help with diagnosis, but the results aren't specific to Behcet's disease. For example, your doctor could perform a **pathergy test**, where a sterile saline solution is injected under the skin; an alternate method is to simply prick the skin of the forearm with a needle. If a pustule [a small elevation of skin filled with lymph or pus] or a nodule develops at the site within 24 to 48 hours, it's a positive reaction, and is very suggestive of a Behcet's diagnosis. The frequency of positive reactions is higher in Mediterranean and Middle Eastern countries[6] than it is in Western countries such as the U.K.[7] or U.S.; however, the test is valid in any part of the world. Other factors can also influence pathergy test results: cleaning the forearm with a disinfectant other than alchohol can reduce the number of positive reactions;[8] and the size of the needle used for the test can significantly impact the results.[9,10] Turkish researchers found that larger, more blunt needles of 0.9 mm diameter (20G), created a higher number of positive results and a more intense reaction than the standard 0.3 mm diameter (26G) disposable needles commonly used today.

In 1991, Cakir reported that injecting patients with **monosodium urate crystals** suspended in saline, instead of injecting with saline solution alone, created a pathergy response more specific to Behçet's disease than to any other rheumatic disease.[76] In a follow-up Turkish study, Fresko (2000) found that the monosodium urate pathergy test created higher levels of positive results in his patients than pricking their forearms three times with a 16G needle. In this study, 97% of patients had a positive pathergy response to the urate crystals, while only 28% tested positive using the more-traditional skin-prick method. One year later, researchers performed repeat pathergy tests on all of the subjects. 95% of the "monosodium urate" patients still showed a positive response when they were injected with the crystals, while 73% of the patients who had their arms pricked in the traditional manner showed a positive response.[105]

In an interesting development, Pickering (2000) suggests caution in the interpretation of Mantoux test results when dealing with Behçet's patients.[22] He discussed an Egyptian BD patient who was given a tuberculin Mantoux skin test, which indicated that the patient had tuberculosis when he actually did not. The patient's health was closely watched over a period of time, and he showed none of the clinical signs or symptoms of TB. He was eventually given a monosodium urate crystal pathergy test; this test caused an abnormal skin response and confirmed the presence of Behçet's, when viewed in combination with his other BD-related symptoms.

In another variation on the pathergy test, Shaquie, Al-Araji and Hatem (2000) performed two types of pathergy tests at the same time, on 25 Iraqi Behçet's patients.[87] One test was the standard prick test on the forearm of each patient; Shaquie also performed **oral pathergy tests** on the inside mucous membrane of each patients' lower lip. A 20G needle was used to prick the skin of the mouth or forearm. The oral test was positive if any ulceration developed at the site, with or without a pustule. Shaquie's study found that the results of oral vs. traditional pathergy tests were similar. The oral test was positive in 56% of the patients, while the standard arm prick test was positive in 60% of the patients. Results of both types of tests were negative in all 29 healthy (non-Behçet's) subjects.

HLA blood testing can also help in diagnosis, although patients need to understand that the results are not specific to Behçet's disease, the test is expensive, it may not be covered by health insurance, and the final report can take weeks to arrive. HLA stands for human leukocyte antigen. HLA types are inherited from both parents. HLA testing is used most often to see if organ donors and organ recipients are compatible, and it is also used for paternity tests and genetic counseling. Research over several decades has shown that HLA-B5 is found more often in the blood of Behçet's patients in Japan, Italy, Korea and Turkey, than in healthy people.[11] Zouboulis (1999) states that HLA-B51 (a split of B5) presents a high risk for Behçet's disease in "a small geographic area of the Mediterranean Sea countries and Southern Asia."[146] HLA-Bw51, HLA-Bw52, HLA-B5101, and HLA-DRw3 have also been implicated in Behçet's studies from various countries[11,14,40]. *[JZ: The **w**, found in HLA-Bw51, for example, was introduced in 1972 by the WHO Nomenclature Committee, and indicated a "temporary" designation. With only a few exceptions, this **w** designation is no longer in use. For our purposes, Bw51, Bw52 and DRw3 can be considered the same as B51, B52 and DR3.[163]]* Other research has raised questions of the relationship between HLA-A2 and DQ3, and the development of Behçet's in some patients;[189] a review by Calamia et al (2000) adds HLA-DR13, DRB1 and DR4 to the mix.[190] An older study by Lehner et al in 1979 indicated that HLA-B5 may be associated more frequently with ocular Behçet's; HLA-B27 may be associated with arthritic symptoms in the absence of rheumatoid arthritis or Reiter's; and B12 is tied to mucocutaneous (skin) involvement.[205,207] It also appears that HLA-DR1 and HLA-DQw1 may confer a certain degree of protection from the development of BD, as these HLA types appear less frequently in patients with Behcet's.[200]

There is apparently no relationship between HLA results and Behçet's disease for patients in the US[12] and the UK[13]. It should be noted, however, that a patient's ethnic background is more important in HLA typing than whether s/he is a resident of a Western country. [221]

While blood for an HLA test is drawn in the same way as standard blood tests, the HLA blood sample is usually forwarded to a specialized lab for processing. Your doctor may request that the lab produce results for HLA-A, HLA-B, HLA-C and/or HLA-D types. Your test results will arrive showing all of the requested HLA types that appear in your blood. For example, my doctor asked for HLA-A and HLA-B tests to be performed, and my report showed the following:

HLA AB Type: A2, A23(9); B7, B50(21)
HLA-C and HLA-D testing was not performed.

The HLA types that appear on your test results will never change during your lifetime, just as your blood type (A, B, AB or O) always stays the

tell from my test results that I don't carry any of the
…es that are common to Behçet's disease. However,
studies mention the possible involvement of HLA-A2
…mal cases of BD, which is a situation that may apply in my
case.[189,191]

**What does all of this HLA lingo mean to me, as a Behçet's
patient?** It means that there's much more to a Behçet's diagnosis than
a simple test. If you have an HLA blood test that shows **HLA-B5, B51,
B5101, or DR3**, there is a higher probability that Behçet's will be your
diagnosis, than if those results hadn't shown up. Lee (2001), gives a
general idea of the odds with the following statement: "In humans,
Behçet's disease occurs in only 1 of 1000 individuals who have the HLA-
B51 phenotype."[188] However, you don't have to show *any* of these HLA
types in order to be diagnosed with Behçet's: physicians base a diagnosis on a combination of observed physical signs and symptoms, their
own personal experience in treating Behçet's patients, the patient's
medical history, and the patient's test results.

Just to complicate the picture further, recent research has
shown that the MICA gene may[15,16] or may not[77,78] also cause a genetic
susceptibility to Behçet's disease — although evidence still seems to lean
more strongly to HLA-B51 as the primary genetic association over any
other potential marker.[79]

**I have Behçet's, and I also tested positive for HLA-B51. I was
told that I'll have a worse case of Behçet's than a BD patient
who doesn't test positive for HLA-B51. Is this true?**
The latest research provides conflicting results on this issue. Gul et al
(2001) looked at 148 Turkish Behçet's patients who had symptoms
lasting for at least five years. The patients were put into groups based
on whether they had mild, moderate, or severe disease activity. Even
though certain symptoms occurred more frequently in the B51-positive
patients (genital ulcerations, skin lesions, positive skin pathergy tests,
and eye disease), there was no connection between being B51-positive
and having a more severe form of Behçet's.[225] Research by Alballa et al
in Saudi Arabia offered a similar conclusion back in 1993.[162] However, a
2001 Korean study by Chang, Kim, Cheon et al provided a comparative
look at 61 Behçet's patients, vs. 56 patients with recurrent aphthous
ulcers, vs. 70 healthy subjects. The researchers concluded that BD
patients with HLA-B51 seemed to be susceptible for uveitis, erythema
nodosum, and the development of "full-blown" [severe] Behçet's.[168]
This result corresponds to Zouboulis' similar 1999 conclusion in
Germany, that being HLA-B51 positive *is* a marker of a more severe
prognosis.[146]

My HLA results aren't any of the ones connected with having Behcet's. Does this mean that I might have some other disease?

Possibly, although as mentioned above, it's not necessary to have a specific HLA result in order to be diagnosed with BD. Only your doctor can help interpret your HLA results in light of your other symptoms or health issues. However, researchers have found that some HLA types do appear more frequently in patients with specific diseases. Some of these disease associations are listed below. If any of your HLA type(s) appear on this list, though, ***do not assume*** that you will develop that particular disease! Please speak with your doctor about any questions you may have on this subject.

<u>**HLA and Disease Associations**</u>

Acute anterior uveitis	B27
Alopecia areata	DR4, DR11, DQB1
Ankylosing spondylitis	B27
Birdshot retinochoroidopathy	A29
Celiac disease	B8, DR3, DQB1, DQA1, DR7, DR11
Dermatitis herpetiformis	DR3
Grave's disease	DR3
Goodpasture's syndrome	DR2
Hashimoto's thyroiditis	DR11
Hemochromatosis	A3
Hodgkin's disease	A1, DRB1
Idiopathic Addison's	DR3
Insulin-dep. diabetes	DR2, DQB1, DR3, DR4, DRB1, DRB5
Juvenile chronic arthritis	B27
Kawasaki disease	B54 (Japanese pts. only)
	B51 (Caucasian pts.)
Lyme disease arthritis	DRB1
Multiple sclerosis	A3, DR15 (a split of DR2), DRB1, DRB5, DQB1
Myasthenia gravis	DR3, B8
Narcolepsy	DR2, DQ1, DW2, DRB1
Optic neuritis	DR15 (a split of DR2)
Pemphigus vulgaris	DR4, DRB1, DQB1
Pernicious anemia	DR11
Polymyalgia rheumatica and giant cell arteritis	DR4
Post-partum thyroiditis	DR4
Presumed ocular histoplasmosis	B7
Psoriasis	B13, Cw6
Reiter's disease	B27
Retinal vasculitis	A29, B8, B44
Rheumatoid arthritis	DR4
Sarcoidosis	B8, DR3
Sicca syndrome	DR3

Systemic lupus erythematosus (SLE)	B8, DR3
Takayasu arteritis	B52 (Japanese patients only)
Uveitis in JRA	high risk=DR5 and DP2 positive, plus DR1 negative

This list should not be considered complete. The most comprehensive listing, with hundreds of possible disease associations, can be found in Tiwari and Terasaki's 1985 Springer-Verlag publication, *HLA and Disease Associations*.

The above HLA disease list was compiled from the following sources:

1) Pile KD. Broadsheet number 51: HLA and disease associations. Pathology 1999 (31), 202-212

2) Thomson G. HLA disease associations: models for the study of complex human genetic disorders. Crit Rev Clin Lab Sci 1995;32(2):183-219

3) Svejgaard A, et al. Associations between HLA and disease with notes on additional associations between a "new" immunogenetic marker and rheumatoid arthritis. In "HLA and Disease: The Molecular Basis." Munksgaard, Copenhagen (1997), p301-13.

4) Friedmann A. "HLA and dermatological disease: Behçet's disease." In "HLA in Health and Disease (2nd Ed)," Lechler and Warrens (Eds.) Academic Press (2000), p372-374

If there are no blood tests or lab tests to diagnose Behçet's, then how *is* it diagnosed?

The diagnosis of Behçet's disease is based on displaying a specific set of physical signs and symptoms, which needs to be recognized and interpreted correctly by the health care provider(s) in charge of your care. These symptoms are listed on page 12, under the heading *International Criteria for Behçet's Disease*. However, it's not necessary to show all of the diagnosable medical problems of BD at the same time, in one office visit. Behçet's may start with just one or two small symptoms that come and go (usually ulcerations), and then other symptoms or clues may appear gradually over the years. Because BD can affect so many different body systems, patients tend to see a variety of specialists, none of whom may be aware of the "big picture" at first. As a result, it might actually take several years before all of the clues are put together and a diagnosis of Behçet's is reached. It's not unusual to hear of patients waiting ten or more years for a BD diagnosis. That's why medical documentation of symptoms, as they appear, is very important. In the event that you can't be seen by a doctor before your current symptoms fade, personal documentation (for example, photographs of skin lesions, or a daily record of health problems) can be helpful for future reference.

Even though there are no tests that will definitely diagnose a case of Behçet's, **certain test results can appear more frequently in BD patients. However, <u>NONE</u> of the results listed on the next page is specifically required for diagnosis.**

Lab test results that appear more frequently in BD patients, usually during times of active disease. NOT required for diagnosis):

1) neutrophil and platelet counts may be increased[80]
2) C-reactive protein (CRP) and ESR may be elevated, and may correlate w/disease activity[81] [O'Duffy (1997) states that it is possible to have active disease (i.e.uveitis) when serum and ESR levels are normal[117]]
3) ANCA, ANA, and antiphospholipid antibodies are usually absent[80]
4) lesions may show a mixed leukocytic infiltration of neutrophils and mononuclear cells into tissues[80,], evidence of cutaneous leukocytoclastic vasculitis[98] or frank necrotizing vasculitis[117]
5) serum immunoglobulins, especially IgA, may be elevated[82]. IgA, IgG and IgM levels may show nonspecific elevations in active neuro-Behçet's.[117]
6) circulating immune complexes (CIC) may be elevated, and may be related to disease activity[85]
7) C3 levels in the cerebrospinal fluid tend to be elevated[83]
8) C9 serum levels may also be elevated[83]
9) clotting time, bleeding time, prothrombin time, and partial thromboplastin time tend to be normal[84]
10) fibrinogen levels may be elevated, and may parallel disease activity[84]
11) IL-8 serum levels may be increased in patients with active oral and neurological symptoms[86]
12) serum amyloid A, and beta-2 microglobulin levels may elevated, and may closely parallel disease activity (Aygunduz et al, 2000, found these tests to be even more sensitive than ESR and CRP levels) [108]
13) rheumatoid factor (RF) may be present, regardless of disease activity[88,89]

What are the *International Criteria for Behçet's Disease*?
The *International Criteria for Classification of Behçet's Disease* were adopted in 1989, at the Fifth International Conference on Behçet's Disease. They are symptoms that are most likely to indicate a case of Behçet's, in the absence of any other medical explanations. The originators recommended that the symptom list be known as "classification" criteria rather than "diagnostic" criteria — they felt that the list was more useful as a way to group patients for Behçet's research studies, rather than as a way to diagnose individual cases of BD.[165] However, because of a lack of laboratory tests specific for Behçet's, and with limited clinical experience in treating BD patients, many physicians lean heavily on the *International Criteria* to help with diagnosis.

Chapter 1

International Criteria for Classification of Behçet's Disease[166]

Recurrent oral ulcerations *[JZ: necessary in ALL cases, in this criteria]*	Minor aphthous ulceration Major aphthous or herpetiform ulceration observed by a physician or reported reliably by patient. Recurrent at least three times in one 12-month period

Plus TWO of the following:

Recurrent genital ulcerations	Recurrent genital aphthous ulceration or scarring, especially males, observed by physician or reliably reported by patient
Eye lesions	a. Anterior uveitis b. Posterior uveitis c. Cells in vitreous on slit lamp examination **or** d. Retinal vasculitis observed by qualified physician (ophthalmologist)
Skin lesions	a. Erythema-nodosum-like lesions observed by physician or reliably reported by patient b. Pseudofolliculitis c. Papulopustular lesions **or** d. Acneiform nodules consistent with Behçet's disease observed by a physician, and in post-adolescent patients not receiving corticosteroids
Positive pathergy test	An erythematous papule, >2mm, at the prick site 48 hr after the application of a sterile needle, 20-22 gauge, which obliquely penetrated avascular skin to a depth of 5mm: read by physician at 48 hr.

Can you be diagnosed with Behçet's and *not* have the necessary symptoms listed above?
Yes. This can happen if a physician is very familiar with the diagnosis and treatment of Behçet's, and understands the relative importance of other serious, unlisted symptoms that the patient may be experiencing.[179] One paper by Lueck et al (1993) described a patient with uveitis and widespread CNS involvement, who was diagnosed with neurosarcoidosis. After the patient's death, an autopsy discovered microscopic tissue changes that indicated a Behçet's diagnosis after all, even though the patient had never suffered from oral or genital ulcerations or arthritic pain.[180] So it is possible (but rare) for a patient to have Behçet's without the hallmark oral ulcers. Unfortunately, at the opposite end of the spectrum, some physicians who are unfamiliar with BD have been known to base a Behçet's diagnosis on nothing more than a single bad case of mouth ulcers.

Are there other lists of Behçet's symptoms besides the
International Criteria?
Yes, there are at least six other Behçet's criteria lists, originating from
various countries around the world. Each list tends to highlight BD
symptoms that the originators feel are important in their specific geographic areas. While the *International Criteria* are generally used to
classify research subjects for Behçet's studies, individual doctors may
choose any one of the criteria lists to help them diagnose their patients.
According to Lee (2001), however, the *International Criteria* have one
specific drawback — the requirement that patients show recurrent oral
ulcers before receiving a Behcet's diagnosis. In his book, ***Behçet's Dis-***
ease: A Guide to its Clinical Understanding, Lee lists several studies
where BD patients have shown no oral symptoms; this situation may delay
proper diagnosis and treatment. He therefore suggests that two diagnostic
criteria be used by physicians at the same time, to compensate for draw-
backs inherent in any one specific set of criteria. Lee's recommendation is
for use of the *International Criteria*, in combination with the revised
(1987) criteria of the Behçet's Syndrome Research Committee of Japan[167] :

Diagnostic Criteria of the
Behçet's Syndrome Research Committee of Japan (1987)

Major symptoms	Recurrent aphthous ulceration of the oral mucous membrane
	Skin lesions
	Erythema nodosum
	Subcutaneous thrombophlebitis
	Folliculitis, acne-like lesions
	Cutaneous hypersensitivity
	Eye lesions
	Iridocyclitis
	Chorioretinitis, retinouveitis
	Definite history of chorioretinitis or retinouveitis
	Genital ulcers
Minor symptoms	Arthritis without deformity and ankylosis
	Gastrointestinal lesions characterizedby ileocaecal ulcers
	Epididymitis
	Vascular lesions
	Central nervous system symptoms
Diagnosis	Complete: Four major features
	Incomplete: Three major features
	or: two major and two minor
	or: typical ocular symptom and one major or two minor features
	Suspected: Two major features or: one major and two minor features

13

What is the "Classification Tree for the Diagnosis of Behçet's Disease"?

The *Behçet's Disease Classification Tree* was created by Davatchi et al in Iran in 1993.[208] They (and some other researchers) consider it to be a more reliable means of diagnosing Behçet's than any of the other major types of diagnostic/classification criteria described above. The *Classification Tree* is a type of flow chart, where yes/no answers to each symptom leads farther down the tree - either stopping at a "non-Behçet's" conclusion, or continuing on to a confirmed Behçet's diagnosis. More information on the *Classification Tree* can be found on page 102.

What kind(s) of doctors should I see if I have Behçet's?

It can be very frustrating finding a doctor familiar with treating Behçet's disease. Many patients must travel to university medical centers or large teaching hospitals to receive appropriate care. Because Behçet's is classified as a rheumatic disease, a rheumatologist may be best qualified to serve as your primary care physician, and as the coordinator of your visits to other health care providers. Your list of specialists may include a neurologist, dermatologist, gastroenterologist, cardiologist and an ophthalmologist, among others.

An ophthalmologist is a necessary member of your treatment team, regardless of how well you are able to see right now. While you may never have any Behçet's-related eye problems in your lifetime, the possibility of visual complications still exists and should be taken seriously. Some retinal complications may be "silent" (non-symptomatic) in the early stages, so it's an important precaution to schedule yearly visits with your ophthalmologist, who will do a full retinal exam each time you're seen. If you start to experience extreme sensitivity to light; hazy, blurred or double vision; new floaters or a sudden increase in floaters; redness around the iris (colored part) of your eye; "blank" or black areas of vision; or severe eye pain, please see your ophthalmologist as soon as possible for evaluation and treatment.

Are there other types of eye problems that can happen to me besides anterior or posterior uveitis, cells in the vitreous, or retinal vasculitis? (all part of the *International Criteria for Behçet's*)

[Definitions in brackets below are from Taber's Cyclopedic Medical Dictionary, 16th Ed.] It's possible to have problems with either the inner or outer parts of the eye, although some complications occur more frequently than others. According to Lakhanpal, O'Duffy and Lie, the following external eye problems have been noted in studies of Behçet's patients: conjunctivitis, subconjunctival hemorrhage, scleritis [inflammation of the sclera, the white outer covering of the eye], episcleritis [inflammation of an area of the sclera under the conjunctiva (lid)], corneal ulceration, keratitis [corneal inflammation], and skin lesions on the eyelids.[66] Matsuo et al (2002) also reported on conjuncti-

val ulcerations that developed on the inner lids of four out of 152 patients at their Japanese hospital; these lesions appeared at the same time as an increase in the patients' other BD-related symptoms.[181]

Internal eye problems can include retinal, macular and optic disc swelling, changes to the retinal pigment, choroiditis [inflammation of the blood vessel area (choroid) between the sclera and retina], chorioretinitis [inflammation of the choroid and retina], optic papillitis [inflammation of the optic disk], vitreous hemorrhage, necrotizing retinitis, retinal vessel phlebitis or arteritis, and retinal detachment. Long-term complications can include cataract development, glaucoma, and optic atrophy. Papilledema [inflammation and swelling of the optic nerve] without uveitis can occur as a result of pseudotumor cerebri [benign intracranial hypertension]. Retinal and vitreous hemorrhages, retinal degeneration, retinal neovascularization [development of small, abnormal blood vessels in the retina], and hypopyon[66,67] have been noted in research studies, although hypopyon [pus in the front of the eye, trapped between the iris and the cornea] is reported less frequently now than in the past. Optic neuropathy [pathological change in the optic nerves, or the blood supply to them], while rare, has also appeared in some cases of Behçet's.[90,91,92] Akman-Demir et al (1999) found that less than 5% of the neuro-Behçet's patients in his study developed optic neuropathy.[109]

I've only had problems in one of my eyes. Will my other eye stay symptom-free?
Unfortunately, one-sided (unilateral) eye involvement is the exception rather than the rule for BD patients. Chee (1998) states that 95% of patients who have eye involvement will have inflammation in both eyes.[97] However, according to BenEzra (1991), if Behçet's-related eye involvement does occur, severity of the visual symptoms may differ quite a bit in each eye.[93] This means that it's possible to have severely decreased vision in one eye, but still have useful vision in the other, even with active inflammation in both. Some "bilaterally-challenged" patients may also find that that both of their eyes are never actually inflamed at the same time. Plotkin (1988) states that problems may start in one eye only, and then be followed in the next symptom flare-up by inflammation in the second eye. However, involvement of the second eye may also take six years or longer to develop.[94] A published report by Pivetti-Pezzi (2000) suggests that any diagnosis of eye involvement as unilateral (one-sided) is due to "defective diagnostic procedures," rather than true one-sided eye disease. She found that indocyanine green angiography discovered previously-undetected leakage and lesions in the supposedly unaffected eyes of two patients. Standard fluorescein angiography and slit lamp examinations had failed to uncover these problems.[95]

Am I going to go blind?
Behçet's patients understandably worry about losing their vision.

Blindness can occur in up to 25% of Behçet's cases.[68,96] One Turkish study (Kural, 2000) found a total loss of vision in 39% of their male eye patients after twenty years of illness, and in 14% of their female eye patients.[164] However, Kural felt that these results were evidence of improved treatment for eye complications: she cited a 1986 study where a staggering 75% of the Behçet's eye patients seen at one treatment center were essentially blind after ten years.

Permanent visual loss is most often caused by complications at the back of the eye-as a result of retinal vasculitis, or branch/central vein occlusions [blood vessel blockages], for example. Many ophthalmologists recommend aggressive treatment against eye complications to prevent the possibility of partial or total vision loss. It's important to remember, however, that **some BD patients never have eye involvement of any kind**. Statistics presented earlier in this chapter show that visual problems occur in 47-73% of Behçet's patients, meaning that a minimum of 27% of diagnosed patients may never have visual complications. Regardless, a full yearly eye exam is recommended for **all** BD patients, and it should be performed by a qualified ophthalmologist (not an optometrist or an optician), using a slit lamp. This type of exam is necessary because some retinal damage caused by Behçet's disease can be "silent" - that is, patients may not be aware that serious problems are beginning or progressing, because there are no immediately obvious symptoms.

Am I going to die from Behçet's Disease?

The majority of BD patients have a normal lifespan. According to Orloff (1999), the mortality rate of patients with Behçet's disease is 3-4%,[7] although Kural et al's study in 2000 suggests a higher 6% rate (26 of their 428 Behçet's patients who were followed for twenty years died of complications directly related to BD).[164] Put into perspective, if 14,000 people in the US have Behçet's disease right now, anywhere from 420 to 840 of those patients may eventually die of complications from BD. The remaining 13,000+ patients will die of other causes - including old age. However, it does appear that young male patients may need to be followed more closely. Yazici et al (1996) looked at 152 male and female BD patients over a 10-year period, and found that the mortality rate among 15- to 24-year-old male patients, in particular, was higher than one would expect to see in the general population; it was also higher than any other patient age group.[18] Kural's study came to the same sobering conclusion about young male patients.[164] Yazici did note that all of the patients who died (a total of six men out of 152 men and women in the original study) tended to have more severe disease symptoms at the time they entered the study. The specific causes of death were: pulmonary arterial aneurysm, inferior and superior vena cava syndromes, upper GI hemorrhage, CNS involvement, and cerebrovascular accident. Pulmonary artery aneurysms, vena caval thrombosis, CNS complications, amyloid nephropathy, and one suicide were the causes of death among the patients in Kural's study.[164] In another study by Park et al (1993), the causes of death in seven Behçet's patients (six men and one woman) were: GI bleeding, bowel perforation, superior and inferior vena cava syndrome, aortic regurgitation, cerebrovascular disease, and lung abscess.[19] In a 1999 study by Kidd et al, two out of 35 neuro-Behçet's patients, followed for a median of three years, died of aspiration pneumonia with severe brainstem impairment.[112] The most recent study (Al-Saleh et al, 2000) followed 208 men and women over a twelve-year period in Saudi Arabia. During that time, five men and one woman died (2.9% of the total enrolled patients). The causes of death were: Budd-Chiari syndrome in three cases; pulmonary hemorrhage (one case); superior and inferior vena cava obstruction and sepsis (one case); and cerebrovascular accident in the remaining case.[69]

As the above studies suggest, women do not appear to die from Behçet's complications as frequently as men. In spite of Walsh and Rau's September 2000 study showing that autoimmune disease is a leading cause of death among young and middle-aged women,[20] Behçet's disease does not specifically appear on their accepted list of 24 autoimmune diseases followed for the study. The most frequent causes of autoimmune mortality for women are: rheumatic fever and heart disease, rheumatoid arthritis, multiple sclerosis, systemic lupus erythematosis, and scleroderma. However, glomerulonephritis [a serious form of kidney inflammation] also appears as one of the top six diseases on Walsh and Rau's list, and glomerulonephritis is known to be a complication of Behçet's disease.[21]

In 2000, Dilsen suggested that the ultimate outcome of any case of Behçet's is dependent on whether or not major (vital) organs have been affected. For the purposes of his study, major organs were defined as: eyes, CNS [central nervous system], deep veins, arteries, heart, bowels, lungs, and the presence of amyloidosis [the creation and deposit of amyloid - a starch-like substance - in tissues and organs, especially the liver, spleen and kidneys during some chronic diseases]. He found that vital organ involvement occurred more frequently in patients with the following characteristics: male; age less than 40; disease starting before the age of 25, first symptom is **not** aphthous ulceration; late diagnosis; and lack of treatment.[99]

Neuro-Behçet's (involvement of the central nervous system) has a worse prognosis than many other forms of Behçet's, justifying its inclusion in Dilsen's "poor outcome" list. In 1999, Akman-Demir et al estimated a mortality rate of approximately 11% during a 5-year follow-up period of 200 neuro-BD patients. However, the researchers were able to list certain factors that influenced the ultimate outcome. For example, if a patient had normal CSF (cerebrospinal fluid) results during an acute neuro-BD attack, there was less resulting disability and a more stable disease course in the long term. However, a high cellular and/or protein count, or brainstem-type involvement, usually resulted in a worse prognosis.[138]

According to Wechsler et al (1999), cardiac manifestations [heart problems] can also create serious complications, and a higher-than expected mortality rate. Possible cardiac problems include coronary artery disease, pericarditis [inflammation of the membrane surrounding the heart], myocardiopathy [disease of the middle layer of the walls of the heart], and valve disease, among other difficulties. Wechsler noted that BD-related coronary artery disease can occur even in young patients, first seen as angina or a heart attack; it has a significant 20% mortality rate in the months or years following diagnosis.[145]

Two recent studies advise caution when performing surgery on Behçet's patients for cardiovascular symptoms. In a study by Kwak et al (2000), fifteen cardiac operations were performed on ten patients over six years. Five of the ten patients died of cardiovascular complications following their surgeries, including three who died of bleeding from a false aneurysm at the surgical site. Surgeries included: aortic valve replacements, Ross procedure, cusp replacement of the aortic valve, and Bentall's procedure.[118] Lee et al (2000) followed nine patients who underwent a total of 17 aortic valve replacements. On average, 44% of the patients died within nine months of the surgery. Deaths were caused by heart failure or infection associated with detachment of the prosthetic valve, or because of leakage around the heart valve(s).[119] Authors of these studies strongly urge either the use of immunosuppressive drugs following surgery, or the pre-surgical use of steroids and other medications, to reduce potentially fatal complications.

While amyloidosis [described earlier] occurs in less than 2% of Behçet's patients, it carries a high 50% mortality rate over 1-11 years. Melikoglu (2000) found that peripheral and pulmonary arterial involvement, and arthritis[106] tend to occur more frequently in patients who eventually develop amyloidosis.

And finally, the mortality rate of BD patients who develop acute Budd-Chiari syndrome is 61%.[17] Budd-Chiari syndrome occurs when major veins of the liver are blocked. Orloff's 1999 study states that "Because the prognosis for long survival is quite good in Behçet's disease, early diagnosis of acute Budd-Chiari syndrome is imperative, and prompt treatment by portal decompression [side-to-side portacaval shunt] is indicated."[17]

Can physical or emotional stress cause Behçet's? (And the reverse: Can Behçet's cause psychological problems?)
Many BD patients have found that personal setbacks or too much physical activity can cause a symptom flare. Researchers tend to agree.

Koptagel-Ital et al (1983) interviewed and tested 53 BD patients, and found that the majority of them were under physical and/or emotional stress before their first Behçet's symptoms appeared. The researchers also noted that, in general, their subjects tended to have weak personalities, "disturbed body image, high anxiety, difficulties in social adaptation" and an inability to express and handle their emotions appropriately.[192]

In 1991, Cengiz and Ozkan looked at fifteen Turkish BD patients who had not taken any medications for at least three months.[193] Ten of the fifteen subjects (66%) said that some form of emotional trauma had occurred before the onset of their symptoms. Precipitating events included: involvement in a kidnapping; wife's death; mother's death; marital problems; theft of all savings; economic setbacks; and academic failure. Two-thirds of interviewed patients were depressed, although the researchers felt that the subjects' depression was caused by discomfort and pain directly associated with BD symptoms.

Researchers have also looked at Behcet's patients who were free of neuro or psychological problems prior to participating in their studies. Achiron et al (1993) found that six out of eleven subjects in their study (55%) had abnormal scores on anxiety testing, and that three patients (27%) tested as being mildly depressed.[194] Statistically higher depression and anxiety scores were additionally found in Calikoglu et al's 2001 study.[195]

Dilsen et al's 1993 study of 63 Turkish Behçet's patients had the following results: 76% of subjects experienced a decrease in energy; 49% had a decrease in professional self-confidence; 65% had difficulty coping with their illness; 35% had an increase in their religious beliefs; and 49% had experienced a change in leisure activities due to BD.[196] In addition, a total 55% of patients in the study were depressed, 22% of them severely. There were higher depression scores found in patients who had low levels of education, and in women with the disease. Dilsen felt that the indefinite prognosis of Behçet's, and the various disabilities caused by the disease, created problems in how patients looked at and dealt with their own lives, and with the people around them.

We have spent a while looking at the psychological profile of "typical" BD patients. What about men and women with established neuro-BD, or ones with occasional neurological symptoms? Psych symptoms in these patients may well be caused by lesions in the brain, as part of the disease process itself. In a 1978 study by Yamada et al,[197] psychological difficulties appeared anywhere from one to eight years after the first neurological symptoms. The first of three psychological stages described by Yamada involved a change in, or regression of, the patient's personality: "being childish, shallow, indifferent, careless, rude, slow in action, euphoric, or depressive." The second stage displayed "forced smiling/crying, amnesia, recent memory impairment, and disorder of sleep rhythm." Those patients with occasional psych symptoms tended to have unusual experiences, such as hallucinations, delusions, confusion, delirium, and "twilight state" [a level of con-sciousness where physical actions are subsequently forgotten; seen, for example, in epileptic seizures].

A 1999 report by Oktem-Tanor et al followed a small group of neuro-BD patients for 35.6 +/-23.7 months, to see what mental deficits occurred over that time period. Their twelve subjects displayed "insidi-ous" cognitive deterioration, regardless of the number of neurological flare-ups that took place. The patients also showed these cognitive deficits before any lesions were seen on MRI or CT scans, indicating that neuro-BD patients should receive periodic neuropsychological testing to spot potential problems. Oktem-Tanor suggested that neuro-Behçet's "can be associated with a special pattern of cognitive deficit, especially memory loss and personality change." Memory loss encom-passed delayed recall, and difficulties with the acquisition and storage of information. Personality changes included lack of inhibition, apathy, and/or attention deficit disorder.[198]

And finally, Farah et al (1998) presented a short report on 41 BD patients, with an emphasis on neurological problems. Twenty-four of the 41 patients had neurological-type symptoms; five of the neuro-BD patients (12% of the original 41 subjects) showed psychological deficits: one had progressive dementia after several strokes; one was severely depressed; one was acutely psychotic; and two exhibited sociopathic behavior [an anti-social personality, with disregard for the rights of others].[199]

Why do my eyes and mouth feel so DRY ?
Some Behçet's patients may be bothered by excessive dryness in the mouth and eyes. Women may also be bothered by vaginal dryness. While only a health care professional can diagnose the cause of these problems, dry eyes in particular may be a side effect of some medica-tions, or may occur as a result of menopause. Some other factors can also cause eye dryness, such as hot, arid or windy climates, high altitudes, air conditioning, Parkinson's disease, thyroid conditions, and Vitamin A deficiencies.[221] Excessive dryness may also be a result of Sjogren's (SHOW grens) syndrome. Sjogren's is an autoimmune disease that can sometimes occur along with other rheumatic diseases, includ-ing Behçet's.[226]

It's important for mouth and eye dryness to be investigated, so that the chance of future complications is reduced. For example, a reduction in saliva can eventually cause an increase in tooth decay, especially along the gumline, as well as increased difficulty in chewing and swallowing. Excessively dry eyes may cause redness, pain, sensitiv-ity to sunlight, and excess mucous accumulation; it may also lead to the creation of ulcers and dry spots on the cornea, which can ultimately affect your vision.[160]

There are medications available to address the various prob-lems associated with Sjogren's. These treatments include Biotene; "Dry Mouth Relief "by Natrol; artifical tears, lubricating ointments, or punctal plugs for dry eyes; and products such as Astroglide for vaginal dryness.

More information on Sjogren's can be found by contacting the Sjogren's Syndrome Foundation, 333 North Broadway, Jericho, NY 11753, www.sjogrens.com; or the National Sjogren's Syndrome Association, 5815 N. Black Canyon Hwy, Phoenix, AZ 85015-2200, www.sjogrens.org.

My hands and feet seem <u>really</u> sensitive to the cold. Does this happen to anyone else?
Yes. You may have Raynaud's (ray NODES) phenomenon. Raynaud's phenomenon can cause your hands, feet, or other parts of the body to become painful, feel "prickly" and/or numb in the cold, and makes them change color temporarily to white or blue. This color change happens because the blood vessels in these areas are overly sensitive to the cold and tend to constrict [narrow], which keeps blood from easily flowing through them. The affected hands or feet may feel cool to the touch. Once these areas start to warm up and blood begins to flow again, it can cause sensations ranging from tingling or throbbing,[161] to extreme pain.

Some people have Raynaud's as their *primary* health issue, while others may have it in addition to Behçet's disease or other rheumatic disorders. When Raynaud's appears in combination with other illnesses, it is referred to as *secondary* Raynaud's.

Treatment for Raynaud's is primarily preventive: make sure to wear warm clothes when going outside in cold weather, and warm your hands or feet slowly if they start to show signs of decreased blood flow. Personal experience has shown the effectiveness of chemically-activated glove inserts such as "Mini-Mini" Hand Warmers, found in many US sporting goods stores (or online at www.grabberwarmers.com). You may also wish to speak with your doctor about drugs that can help ease your symptoms. The National Institute of Health (www.nhlbi.nih.gov) states that vasodilators can relax blood vessel walls to improve blood flow through the affected areas.

Additional Raynaud's information can be found through the Arthritis Foundation, (www.arthritis.org) 1314 Spring Street, Atlanta, GA 30309; phone: (404) 872-7100.

What can you tell me about mouth ulcers?
Many undiagnosed Behçet's patients have been told to accept their painful mouth ulcers, because "everyone gets canker sores." Indeed, aphthous ulcers appear commonly in the mouths of 5-25% of the general population;[158] often, the cause of these sores is never found. However, some possible reasons for recurrent aphthous mouth ulcers (besides Behçet's disease) can be: a vitamin B1, B2, B6, or B12 deficiency; an allergy to sodium lauryl sulfate in toothpaste; gluten or other food sensitivity; deficiencies in folic acid, iron, selenium or zinc; viral or bacterial causes (e.g. herpes simplex or streptococcal infections); or as a

result of other systemic conditions such as Crohn's disease, ulcerative colitis, HIV/AIDS, MAGIC syndrome, Reiter's syndrome, or SLE (systemic lupus erythematosus).[65] Rogers (2001) cites studies that implicate preservatives and dyes such as cinnamaldehyde, benzoic acid, sorbic acid, and azo dyes.[218]

In the same way that a cold sore announces its impending arrival, the place where an aphthous ulcer is going to appear often itches, burns or stings in advance. A reddish patch then develops at the site, and evolves into a shallow ulceration covered by a yellow-white or tan membrane; the entire ulcer is circled by a reddish halo. This ulcer may deepen, or meet up with adjoining ulcers to create a larger inflamed area.

There are different categories of mouth ulcers depending on their severity, the frequency of recurrence, and the sheer number of sores appearing at any one time:[218,219]

Recurrent aphthous stomatitis (RAS) is another name for canker sores. RAS is divided into two main categories: simple aphthosis, and complex aphthosis.

Simple RAS: These mouth ulcers may occur anywhere from three to six times per year, and they tend to heal quickly, with limited amounts of pain and disability.

Complex RAS: In comparison to "simple" ulcerations, complex mouth sores have the potential to be very disabling. They can cause a great deal of pain, be slow to heal, and in some cases they can be relentless, with new ulcers forming even as old ones heal.

Aphthous mouth ulcers can also be classified as minor, major, or herpetiform.

Minor ulcerations: These painful sores tend to be small (3-10 mm in size), occur in sets of one to five lesions per flare, and generally heal within 7-14 days. They appear in the mouths of 75-85% of canker sore sufferers, and may be located in the following areas: the inside cheeks, inside of the lips, the front top and bottom of the tongue, the floor of the mouth, and the soft palate (the soft area of the roof of the mouth, by the throat). While rare, ulcerations may also occur on the hard palate, the gums, the rear of the tongue, and the lips themselves. These canker sores usually start in childhood or adolescence, and have a highly variable recurrence rate: anywhere from one or two times per month, to once every several months or years.

Major ulcerations: Major ulcerations tend to be larger (1-3 cm) and deeper than the minor aphthous ulcers described above. As a result, they can take much longer to heal - approximately two to six weeks - and often leave scars. Ten to 15% of people with RAS have these major sores, which can be accompanied by fever, sizable amounts of pain, and an overall sick feeling. Major ulcerations can occur anywhere in the mouth, but the inside of the lip(s), soft palate, and tonsil area are favored locations.

Herpetiform ulcerations: Despite the name, herpetiform ulcers are **not** caused by the herpes simplex virus. Only 5-10% of patients with RAS (usually young women) experience this ulcerative form, which creates the largest number of lesions per episode: sores can be grouped in any amount, usually from ten to 100 at a time. These sores are small but mighty, as individual lesions can merge with adjacent ones to form larger and deeper ulcerated areas. Healing may take one to four weeks, and often results in scarring. In severe cases, persistent or destructive aphthous ulcers may require surgical intervention.

What treatments or medications can help my mouth ulcers?

Please Note: The information provided below is meant to support, and not replace, the relationship that exists between a patient and his/her health care provider. Please speak with your doctor before making any changes to your treatment plan. That advice includes trying any of the products listed here. Some of these medications help with the pain of oral ulcers; some speed healing. All of these medications have been suggested by individual Behçet's patients, their physicians, and/or as a result of searches through medical literature. The listing of specific trade names does not imply endorsement of those particular products over any others.

Over-the-counter (OTC) treatments: Carmex ointment, medicated Blistex, Orabase, Ambesol, Dr. Tichenor's mouthwash diluted 3:1, Listerine mouthwash, raspberry leaf tea, toothpastes with baking soda and peroxide, CloSYSII toothpaste or mouthwash, Rembrandt toothpaste (does not containsodium lauryl sulfate, which has been linked to canker sores), or Zilactin.

Prescription-only, local anesthetics (numbs ulcerated areas short-term to allow for eating): TOPEX (20% benzocaine gel; single-dose anesthetic swabs, metered spray, or flavored liquid), Lidocaine Viscous 2%, Zetacaine (used by dentists to numb mouth before Novocaine injection), Hurricaine topical anesthetic, Lidex (fluocinonide) gel 0.05%.

Prescription-only, medications to help in healing of current ulcerations: Aphthasol (amlexanox) 5% paste, Kenalog (triamcinolone acetonide) in Orabase, Peridex mouth rinse, PerioGard, Difflam mouth rinse (benzydamine hydrochloride 0.15%), Corsodyl (chlorhexidine gluconate 0.2%), Tetracycline rinse (250mg capsules dissolved in 10ml of water; hold in the mouth for 3 minutes and spit out.)

Prescription systemic medications: Colchicine, Trental (non-generic version strongly recommended over generic pentoxifylline), Dapsone, Ergamisol (levamisole hydrochloride), Prednisone/Prednisolone, Thalidomide.

This is only a partial list of mouth ulcer treatments. There is a comprehensive review of different therapies for mouth ulcers and other oral problems contained in the **Treatments** *chapter of this book.*

That's a lot of options. How do I know which one is right for me?
Drugs that work for one patient's symptoms might not help another
patient at all. You and your doctor may need to use a trial-and-error
approach before finding the proper drug or combination of treatments
that works best in your situation.

Many doctors employ a "stepladder" approach when choosing
medications to treat Behçet's symptoms. This means that the treatments with the lowest overall body impact will be tried first. If those
treatments don't work, or create unacceptable side effects, your doctor
will move up to the next rung of the ladder. For example, if your mouth
ulcers are sporadic and not too disabling, topical medications or oral
rinses may work best. If those options don't provide sufficient relief, it is
possible to inject steroids directly into the ulcer(s).

For people with more frequent sores, Trental (the brand name
of generic pentoxifylline) is a good next step. Taken orally at 400 mg
three times per day, Trental can help to reduce or eliminate oral and
genital ulcers; it can also assist with joint pain and fatigue. However,
Trental may take up to three months to reach its full effect. It is important to know that, for many BD patients, the generic version of Trental
does not work as well as the name brand. Additional possibilities for
treatment include colchicine or Dapsone. Thalidomide is used as a last
resort due to its potential for creating birth defects and irreversible nerve
damage - but for some patients with relentless and incapacitating ulcers,
Thalidomide can open the door to a new life.

Moderate-to-high doses of prednisone can temporarily beat
back a severe case of ulcerations, while the patient begins alternate
long-term treatment. Due to its serious side effects when taken for long
periods, however, prednisone should always be tapered, and then
discontinued, as soon as possible.

**I've heard that there's something called "Magic Mouthwash"
that might help my mouth ulcers. What is it?**
__Magic Mouthwash__ is an oral rinse that can be created by your
pharmacist, with a prescription from your doctor. It can help with pain
relief, and also helps ulcers to heal faster. This is the recipe:

> 28cc Mylanta
> 30cc Viscous Xylocaine
> 30cc Benadryl liquid
> 30cc Nystatin
> 2cc Hydrocortisone/Wydase
> *Swish with 5-10cc before meals, and as needed, for pain relief.*

__Bilson's Solution__ is a similar type of mixture, also requiring a
prescription:

> 2gm tetracycline (4x500mg caps)
> 60cc Nystatin Suspension
> 100mg hydrocortisone pdr. q.s.
> 240cc Diphenhydramine Elixir
> *Gargle/swish, then swallow 15cc four times per day.*

And finally, there are two recipes that can be made at home-but be sure to check with your doctor before using either of them:

> One part liquid Benadryl
> Two parts liquid antacid (such as Mylanta)
> Add just a little water
> *Swish/gargle and hold in mouth as long as possible, then swallow (or spit out if you don't want Benadryl to make you sleepy). Use twice a day, with one additional dose before bed.*

One dentist suggested using equal parts of Mylanta and Benadryl, instead of a 2:1 ratio.

What can I use to treat external genital swelling, inflammation, and ulcerations?

Please Note: The information provided below is meant to support, and not replace, the relationship that exists between a patient and his/her health care provider. Please speak with your doctor before making any changes to your treatment plan. That advice includes trying any of the products listed here. Some of these medications help with the pain of genital ulcers; some speed healing. All of these medications have been suggested by individual Behçet's patients, their physicians, and/or as a result of searches through medical literature. The listing of specific trade names does not imply endorsement of those particular products over any others.

Numbing agents: Vagisil; Baby Orajel (use with a covering of Vaseline prior to urinating); Lidocaine Viscous 2%; Instillagel (clinimed) — an anesthetic and antiseptic; ELA-Max 5 (5% lidocaine); Sustaine Blue Gel (works on broken skin only; contains lidocaine, tetracaine and epinephrine); Liquidcaine (4% lidocaine for broken skin areas; non-stinging, deadens in 90 seconds); EMLA cream.

Topical preparations to relieve inflammation and swelling, and aid in healing: Preparation H or similar hemorrhoidal products; Lidex (fluocinomide); Bactroban (mupirocin); Sigmacort (hydrocortisone acetate); Kenacomb cream/ointment (nystatin, neomycin base, gramicidin, and triamcinolone); Mycolog cream/ointment (nystatin and triamcinolone); Elocon cream (mometasone furoate); Peridex applied genitally; Kenalog paste; Bag Balm.

Prescription systemic medications: Colchicine; Trental (non-generic version); Dapsone; Ergamisol (levamisole hydrochloride); prednisone/prednisolone; Cyclosporine; interferon alpha-2A; Thalidomide; Imuran; CellCept; Enbrel; Remicade.

Where do Behçet's-related genital sores appear?
Aphthous ulcerations can appear on the scrotum, vulva, prepuce
[foreskin of the penis], glans penis [bulbous end of the penis], shaft of
the penis, vagina, exterior vaginal opening, fourchette [a mucous
membrane connecting the posterior ends of the labia minora to the
vagina], cervix, clitoris, urethra, anus, perineum, groin, and buttocks.[63]
While external vulvar lesions may be very painful, cervical and vaginal
ulcerations may not be noticed until painful intercourse uncovers the
problem, and/or until the lesions produce a discharge. According to
Zouboulis (2000), perigenital [around the genitals] and anal aphthous
ulcerations are found more often in pediatric Behçet's patients than in
adult patients.[67]

**I always seem to get genital ulcers (and other BD symptoms)
right before my period. Is this a coincidence?**
No. Many women with Behçet's find that their symptoms increase
immediately before or during their menstrual periods due to hormonal
factors.[100,101,102] Anyone with this problem might want to discuss the
phenomenon with a gynecologist, as regulating or eliminating hormonal
fluctuations through the use of birth control pills could decrease the
symptoms or flares.[221] Hormonal changes have also been known to
increase symptoms in other autoimmune disorders. For example,
Ostensen et al found that 72% of female patients in their 1997
fibromyalgia (FM) study had a pre-menstrual increase in FM-related
health problems.[103]

**Are aphthous ulcers the only type of genital complications
that you can get with Behçet's?**
No, although aphthous ulcerations are the only genital complications
listed as part of the *International Criteria for Behçet's Disease*. Other
types of genital lesions that have appeared in studies of Behçet's
patients include vesicles [blisterlike elevations on the skin], erythema-
tous macules [discolored spots or patches on the skin, in various colors,
sizes and shapes], papules [red, solid, elevated areas on the skin],
nodules, folliculitis [inflamed hair follicles], and sterile pustules.[63] In
addition, Zouboulis (2000) states that orchitis [inflammation of a
testicle], prostatitis [inflammation of the prostate gland] and ovarian
cysts, while less common, can also appear in cases of BD.[70]

A study by Wilbur, Maurer and Smith (1993) cautions against
the possible misinterpretation of Pap smears from BD patients, especially when a clinical history is not reviewed prior to the report. They
presented the case of a 52-year-old woman whose Pap smear results
suggested a keratinizing squamous cell carcinoma [malignant tumor].
In actuality, she had acute ulcerative lesions in her vagina that were
severely inflamed. The Pap smear had been prepared from a vaginal
rather than cervical sample, because the patient had undergone a

hysterectomy fifteen years previously. As Wilbur states, "The presence of a large amount of obscuring purulent exudates and cellular debris, in such a situation, should give the examiner reason to be cautious in diagnosing squamous cell carcinoma." [107]

I get the same kind of ulcers on other parts of my body that I get in my mouth. Are there any medications that I can use to heal them?

In 1992, Azizlerli published a study describing these "extragenital" aphthous ulcers. They look like oral ulcers, recur like oral ulcers, and may leave scar tissue similar to what is left by many genital ulcers or major oral ulcerations. Approximately 3% of the 970 Behçet's patients in Azizlerli's study had this form of extragenital skin lesion.[61] Extragenital ulcerations were also described in a clinical study by Chen in 1997. He reported that it was possible for patients to have more than one type of Behçet's-related skin lesion at the same time.[62] For example, a patient could have erythema nodosum on her legs, and have simultaneous extragenital ulcers on her scalp and on one breast. Many of these lesions can be treated with topical corticosteroids, such as Sigmacort. In addition, Elocon lotion (mometasone furoate) is one treatment that can be applied directly to scalp lesions. Systemic medications that can help heal skin ulcers include: Colchicine (more helpful in preventing future lesions than healing current ones), Trental (non-generic version of pentoxifylline), Dapsone, Ergamisol (levamisole hydrochloride), prednisone/prednisolone, Cyclosporine, interferon alpha-2A, and Thalidomide.

Sores have also been known to appear within the nostrils, as well as within the folds of the outer ears.

Are there other types of skin lesions that I can get with Behçet's, besides aphthous ulcers?

Yes. The following four types of skin lesions are all listed as part of the *International Criteria for Behçet's disease*[71] [definitions based on Taber's Cyclopedic Medical Dictionary, 16th Ed] :

erythema-nodosum-like lesions [red and painful nodules, usually on legs]

pseudofolliculitis [inflammation of hair follicles, sometimes looking like a rash of whiteheads on the back, shoulders or other areas]

papulopustular lesions [solid, red, flat or elevated areas on the skin, may become filled with pus or lymph]

acneiform nodules [resembling acne; may include cysts and nodules that leave scars].

Researchers have also found other kinds of skin lesions in BD patients: nodules, vesicles [blisterlike elevations on the skin], furuncles [boils], abscesses, pyodermas [acute, pustular bacterial skin inflammations], impetigo [inflammatory skin disease with pustules that crust and rupture], erythema multiforme-like lesions [dark red elevated area(s) on the skin, sometimes appearing in rings], psoriasis, purpura [hemorrhaged areas in the skin, may appear red, darkening into purple; discolored areas do not disappear under pressure], urticaria [e.g. hives], eczema, and paronychia [redness and swelling around the nail edge], among others.[64]

A recent study by Diri et al (2001) indicated that papulopustular skin lesions are seen more often in Behçet's patients who have arthritic symptoms.[206] This study did not include BD patients less than 25 years old, or ones being treated with corticosteroids, in order "to avoid the age and drug-associated acne lesions."

I've been having some awful problems with diarrhea lately, but then sometimes I get constipated instead. I'm not eating or drinking anything different. What's going on?
Make sure to discuss this situation with your doctor, as these problems can be serious. For example, diarrhea can cause dehydration, electrolyte imbalances, and other potentially life-threatening complications. Lee et al (2001) report that gastrointestinal problems affect 4-28% of Behçet's patients;[227] Chung et al (2001) give a higher percentage: 10-50%, depending on where the patient lives.[239] Any part of the GI system may be involved, from the mouth to the rectum. According to Plotkin (1988), the following GI symptoms have been reported in BD patients: "recurrent sore throats, oral fetor [bad breath], referred otalgia [pain felt in the ear, although the origin of the pain is somewhere else in the body], odynophagia [pain upon swallowing] and dysphagia [difficulty in swallowing]-*[JZ: either of which may be caused by oral ulcerations, or by narrowing of the pharynx from ulcerative scar tissue]*, oropharyngeal pain, anorexia, vomiting, flatulence, dyspepsia [imperfect or painful digestion], regurgitation, eructation [belching], retrosternal and abdominal pain *[JZ: including lower right quadrant pain similar to that found in appendicitis]*, abdominal distention [swelling], diarrhea which may be accompanied by mucus and/or blood, constipation, tenesmus [spasms of the anal sphincter, with pain and persistent desire to empty the bowel or bladder], pain on defecation, and anal pain."[235] The salivary glands or parotid gland may become enlarged and/or swollen. In addition, single or multiple lesions may develop in the esophagus: Yashiro et al (1986) described three BD patients with dissection of esophageal mucosa, esophageal ulcers, and esophageal varices.[236]

Kasahara et al (1981) reported on the locations of intestinal ulcers found in 114 patients: the terminal ileum in 44% of the cases; the ileocecal region in 34%; and the cecum in 12%.[237] Some patients had lesions in more than one area. The report also included a description of the less common lesion locations: the ileum, duodenum, transverse colon, ascending colon, stomach, and jejunum. Bayraktar et al (2000), however, noted that the most common areas of GI involvement in their

Turkish patients were the ileocecal region and the colon.[240] Gastrointestinal lesions and their resulting symptoms may become frequent during overall Behçet's flare-ups; however it's also possible for the various GI problems to appear independently of other BD symptoms.[240]

It can be difficult to distinguish the intestinal lesions of Behçet's disease from those of Crohn's or other GI disorders. As noted in a later chapter in this book on the differential diagnosis of BD and Crohn's, based on a study by Chung et al (2001), "The imaging hallmarks of GI-Behçet's are the presence of deep, penetrating or punched-out ulcers, uneven thickening of the bowel wall, and the absence of granulomas (although granulomas are also absent in up to 50% of Crohn's patients). The GI ulcers may create a high number of complications, such as bowel perforation, fistulas, hemorrhage, and peritonitis."[239] Excellent CT and barium image examples of lesions can be seen in Chung et al's **Radiologic findings of Behcet syndrome involving the gastrointestinal tract.** Radiographics 2001;21:911-924.

Finally, Plotkin's 1988 review of GI problems noted that some Behçet's patients with small-bowel involvement may have difficulties with digestion, and with absorption of nutrients.[238] This conclusion was based on research performed by Oshima (1963) and Shimizu (1979). It is interesting to note that two of fifteen patients interviewed for **You Are Not Alone: 15 People with Behçet's** have problems with pseudo-obstruction gastroparesis, also known as delayed emptying, or "motility problems of the smooth muscle tissue."[241] Simply stated, after eating, food remains in the stomach much longer than it should. Patients with this problem often experience nausea and abdominal pain following meals, and sometimes vomit undigested food hours later. Gubbins and Bertch (1991) suggest that when gastric emptying is delayed, it may also cause problems with the absorption of certain drugs taken by patients. In addition, they note that people with inflammatory GI diseases, such as Behçet's and GI-scleroderma, may have drug absorption problems regardless of any motility difficulties.[242]

What treatments can be used for gastroparesis? According to McCallum and George (2001), the following drugs may be helpful: metoclopramide by injection, and low-dose erythromycin-either alone or in combination with metoclopramide. The researchers also encourage the use of anti-nausea medications.[243] However, the new treatment of choice appears to be *gastric pacing:*[244] the surgical installation of a gastric electrical stimulation pacemaker (Forster et al, 2001). Clinical trials from 1998 through 2000 showed a significant lessening of the severity and frequency of nausea and vomiting after three months, an effect that was sustained throughout the twelve-month trial period. In addition, there was an improvement in gastric emptying times and patients' nutritional status, and a decrease in the number of patient hospitalizations.

I've had some urinary problems over the last few weeks. Could this be related to BD?

Involuntary leakage of urine can occur as people age, or may be due to other physiological problems such as a urinary tract infection, urinary sphincter weakness, weak bladder muscles, anatomical changes caused by childbirth, or bladder stones. Emotional disturbances, and some medications (such as narcotics) may also play a part.[60] However, there are some types of urinary problems that can specifically appear in a small percentage of Behçet's patients who have neurological involvement. These problems include difficulty in starting urination, having to urinate more frequently than normal, having a sudden urge to urinate, and incontinence (inability to control urination). A study of 24 Behçet's patients with neurological symptoms (Erdogru et al, 1999) found that 50% of these patients experienced some degree of urinary difficulty.[23] A limited study of eight patients (Cetinel et al, 1999) found higher results, with problems due to either neurological complications or direct bladder involvement. In two of the cases, ulcers or lesions were found in the bladder.[24] However, statistics from these two studies are quite different from Lida's (2000), who said that urinary problems appear in only 5% of patients with neuro-Behçet's.[25] Regardless, Erdogru feels that the neurogenic bladder can be caused by inflammation in the nervous and vascular systems, which should be treated before irreversible damage occurs.[23] Because these kinds of urinary problems can also appear in medical conditions such as multiple sclerosis, patients need to be evaluated carefully.

What about urinary tract infections?

There are several different types of urinary tract infections (UTIs), including infections of the urethra (urethritis) and the bladder (cystitis). Both urethritis and cystitis have been observed in studies of Behçet's patients.[147,148,149]

What is epididymitis?

According to Taber's Medical Dictionary, the epididymis is "a small oblong body...that constitutes the first part of the excretory duct" contained within each testicle. Epididymitis can cause pain and swelling of the epididymis in one or both testicles. According to **Behçet's Disease: A Contemporary Synopsis**, "Epididymitis, which is listed as a minor criterion [of Behcet's disease], presents as a transient swelling with haphalgesia [pain caused by lightly touching the affected area]. Epididymitis may occur with variable frequency, can present as spontaneous painless or painful swelling lasting for one to two weeks, and may be recurrent. Urethroscopic examination in a patient with Behçet's disease and recurrent epididymitis associated with a urethral discharge disclosed aphthous ulcerations of the urethral mucous membrane."[222] Epididymo-orchitis may also occur in male patients.

Orchitis is an inflammation of one or both testicles, accompanied by pain, swelling and fever. According to Assaad-Khalil (1991), "epididymo-orchitis occurred at least once in 50% of our [Egyptian] male patients, and has been recurrent in half of them."[223] In contrast, only 8% of American men in Calamia et al's 2000 study experienced epididymitis.[224]

Can the kidneys be affected?
Kaklamani et al published a case report in 2001, along with a review of the literature concerning Behçet's-related kidney involvement.[169] They concluded that renal involvement in Behçet's can involve the following features: glomerulonephritis [a type of kidney inflammation] - diffuse crescentic, focal and segmental necrotizing; renal vein thrombosis; and amyloidosis. In addition, the following test results can occur: proteinuria [protein in the urine] (20-55%); hematuria [blood in the urine](20-31%); and, on occasion, elevated levels of creatinine.

In their own 2002 study, Akpolat et al came to the following conclusions [202] :

1) Renal involvement in Behçet's is more frequent than previously thought.

2) Male gender is a risk factor for all types of BD-related kidney involvement.

3) Amyloidosis can affect the patient's ultimate survival, and Behçet's patients with vascular involvement have a high risk of developing amyloidosis [a metabolic disorder where amyloid, a starchlike material, is produced and deposited in organs and tissues; the kidneys, spleen and liver are frequently involved]. Colchicine may be helpful for these patients.

In 1999, Apaydin et al demonstrated that it is possible to perform a successful kidney transplant in a Behçet's patient, with none of the post-operative complications seen in other BD-related surgical procedures. They credit their success partly on the extensive use of immunosuppressive and anti-inflammatory medications following the surgery.[201]

I've been having trouble getting (and keeping) an erection.
This problem is called *erectile dysfunction* (impotence), and there are many different reasons that it can happen. For example, some medications can cause impotence, including drugs for treatment of high blood pressure, antidepressants, antipsychotic medications, some sedatives, cimetidine, lithium and alcohol.[58] In the general population, impotence can also have a medical basis such as diabetes, injury to the penis, problems with the penile blood supply, or damage to nerves leading to and from the penis. As men age, impotence becomes more common: about 50% of 65-year-old men, and 75% of 80-year-old men are

impotent. This is usually a result of the various health problems that can affect older people. Impotence in normally healthy, younger men tends to have a psychological basis.[58]

However, it's also possible for erectile dysfunction to be a frustrating problem associated with Behçet's disease, regardless of the patient's age. In addition to the medications listed above, some drugs used to treat BD patients can cause erectile dysfunction. These drugs include cyclophosphamide (Cytoxan), sulphasalazine (Azulfidine), indomethacin (Indocin), naproxen (Naprosyn) and thalidomide (Thalomid).[26] Psychological factors may also come into play: Behçet's patients with genital ulcer experience sometimes have second thoughts about sexual intercourse — especially if the friction of intercourse has caused painful genital lesions in the past. Erdogru found that 63% of the men in his study of neuro-Behçet's patients had some difficulty getting and maintaining an erection. [23] These men ranged in age from 24 to 55 years old. Akman-Demir et al (1999) had similar results, reporting that impotence occurred in more than 50% of their male patients with CNS involvement.[109] Aksu et al (2000) found that even male Behçet's patients without neurological involvement could experience erectile dysfunction. The two [non neuro-BD] patients discussed in his report were not taking any of the problematic drugs mentioned above, and had no other co-existing diseases or infections. Severe venous leak was the cause of their impotence.[26] According to Aksu, since Behçet's is a chronic systemic vasculitis that can take many forms, male patients may unfortunately experience impotence at some point in their illness.

I stopped smoking, and now my mouth is full of ulcers. Is there a connection?

Yes. Researchers have found that smokers tend to have fewer aphthous ulcers in general than non-smokers.[27,28,29,30,41] According to Axell (1985), people who smoke pipes or cigarettes without filters have the most protection against mouth ulcers. This connection also extends - to a lesser degree - to people who use smokeless (chewing) tobacco, snuff, and filtered cigarettes. These findings led researchers to conclude that the nicotine in tobacco products provides protection against mouth ulcers. As a result, nicotine replacement gum (four 2 mg tablets per day) or nicotine patches have been found to prevent ulcerations in the mouths of people who try to stop smoking. Studies have also shown that non-smokers (including ulcerative colitis patients) who have excessive problems with mouth ulcers can be helped through the short-term use of nicotine replacement products. However, long-term use of any of these products is **not safe or recommended.**

In an interesting development, Rizvi and McGrath Jr. (2001) reported on two patients whose use of cigarette smoking appeared to provide systemic relief of oral *and* genital ulcerations.[170] The substitution of a nicotine patch for smoking had no effect on the one patient who tried that option. In addition, one of the two patients found partial or total relief, through smoking, of other BD-related symptoms, including erythema nodosum, inflammatory polyarthritis, pathergy and "subjective neuropsychiatric symptoms." Both Rizvi and McGrath recognize the dangers in promoting cigarette smoking to patients, but suggest that a larger-scale, well-controlled study of this phenomenon may provide useful results for future treatment.

My Behçet's symptoms always seem to get worse in very hot (or cold, or humid, or rainy) weather. Am I imagining this?
No, although most of the evidence for a weather/symptom correlation comes from individual Behçet's patients, rather than scientific studies. Many BD patients, when asked, can easily identify weather patterns or times of the year that are particularly problematic for them. Unfortunately, only three studies were found that mention this phenomenon. In Korea, Bang (1997) looked at 246 Behçet's patients, and found that 21% had symptoms that increased due to seasonal changes. The highest percentage of patients (approx 36%) became worse in the spring, followed by 32.5% in summer and 23.6% in winter. Only 8% of patients experienced more problems in the fall.[37] Cho et al (1991) discovered that almost 30% of the 57 children with Behcet's in their study had seasonal flare-ups of BD symptoms, with the majority of problems coming in the summer.[72] Israeli researchers [31] looked at Behcet's and lupus (SLE) patients' symptoms in relation to temperature, humidity, barometric pressure, and ultraviolet radiation. While SLE patients tended to worsen in the winter (more joint pains, weakness, fatigue, Raynaud's phenomenon, rash, number of hospital admissions, time off from work, and increase in medications), Behçet's patients showed an increase only in joint pains during autumn and spring. This low-key result is unusual, considering research results in other related diseases. Zatorska et al (2000) found a seasonal basis to uveitis in children from 4-18 years old: spring and fall were the most prevalent times for inflammations, with occasional flare-ups at the beginning of summer.[32] Another study followed eight women with fibromyalgia over a period of three months, and found a significant correlation between pain levels, amounts of sleep, and the weather conditions that the women experienced.[33] A study of 92 patients with rheumatoid arthritis found that 34% of patients believed their symptom flares were caused by changes in the weather[34], and patients with multiple sclerosis often notice that high temperatures increase their symptoms.[35]

However, the most recent study on seasonal symptom severity in 1,424 patients with rheumatic diseases (Hawley et al, 2001) attempts to debunk any possible connection between weather and an increase in disease symptoms. Even though almost 50% of the studied patients reported that their levels of pain, fatigue and health complications increased during certain seasons, the researchers found no such connection. Hawley stated that these supposed seasonal differences "reflect perception rather than reality, since reported symptoms do not agree with measured clinical scores."[36]

Can Behçet's disease affect the joints? My right knee hurts for a few days every month, and then the pain goes away. Sometimes my other knee hurts instead, and it swells up.

Yes, arthritis [inflammation of a joint], arthralgia [joint pain] and synovitis [inflammation of the membrane lining the capsule of a joint] are all common in Behçet's, affecting anywhere from 31-79% of BD patients.[227] Children are more likely than adults to experience joint involvement.[228] A retrospective review of 340 BD cases involving joint manifestations was undertaken by Benamour et al (1998) in Morocco. They found that more than half (57%) of the studied patients struggled with joint problems; in 18% of those cases, arthritis and arthralgia were the first BD-associated symptoms that the patients experienced.[228] Pain and/or swelling of the joint(s) may be asymmetrical -- for example, only one knee may be involved at a time - and more than one type of joint may be affected during a symptom flare-up. It appears that knees and ankles are the most commonly-involved joints; other possible sites include wrists, elbows, large limb joints, and the small joints of the hands and feet. Diri et al (2001) found that 27% of his subjects also experienced non-inflammatory low back pain.[206] Patients will most often experience pain, tenderness, swelling, limitation of joint movement, warmth, and morning stiffness.[229] BD-associated arthritis can be either intermittent or chronic.[230] It is usually non-destructive to the affected joints, although Benamour noted polyarthritis with deformities and/or destruction in eight of his patients.[228]

El-Ramahi et al (1993) performed joint aspirations on eight Behçet's patients with arthritis. They found "the range of WBC varied from 1100-17,300 cells/mm³ and PMN predominated (77%). Synovial fluid analysis in BD is useful to exclude infections and crystal deposition causes of arthritis; however, it will not help to differentiate the arthritis of BD from other inflammatory arthritides."[231] A report by O'Duffy et al (1971) described leukocyte counts of 10,000 and 7500 cells/mm³ with PMN of 75% in two joint fluid analyses.[232]

Why am I so tired? My family says I never seem to get off the couch

Fatigue is a common complaint of Behçet's patients. Surprisingly little research has been done on this problem, although 37% of BD patients in a study by Oh et al (1985) reported feelings of fatigue.[131] In 1999, Bhakta et al released their "Behçet's Disease Clinical Activity Form," where fatigue levels are measured as one of several clinical features tracked by physicians. Bhakta readily admits that the underlying cause for fatigue in BD patients is unknown; it may be due to BD itself, or to a co-existing medical condition such as fibromyalgia.[132] Akman-Demir et al have found, though, that 6% of the 200 neuro-Behçet's patients in their 1999 study experienced excessive daytime sleep episodes.[138]

One difficulty comes in determining the patient's own definition of the word fatigue. Is s/he describing muscle weakness, or a "bone-tired" feeling, or is s/he referring to actual sleepiness during the daytime? Is the fatigue possibly related to medicinal side effects, or could it be caused by a specific sleep disorder, depression, or drug/ alcohol abuse?

Regardless, overwhelming fatigue does occur with great frequency in patients who have rheumatic and/or chronic diseases.[133,134] Swain (2000) feels that this common symptom is often ignored by physicians, who would prefer to address concrete and more-easily-treatable health problems in their patients.[134]

In 1996, Wolfe et al looked at 1,488 patients who had a variety of rheumatic diseases. The researchers found that it was possible to predict fatigue levels from the patients' pain and depression levels, from the amount of sleep disturbances that they experienced, and from the number of "tender points" on the body (related to fibromyalgia). Not surprisingly, fatigue was also an accurate predictor of problems at work, as well as a predictor of the patients' overall health status.[135]

As stated above, fatigue may be caused by disruptions in the sleep cycle. According to Shimokawabe et al (1991), past studies have shown that Behçet's can cause problems with the autonomic nervous system (ANS). The ANS regulates heart and breathing rates, blood pressure, body temperature, and other functions that operate without conscious effort. Testing of the autonomic nervous system can be done through sleep studies, which indicate dysfunctional sleep patterns. For example, Shimokawabe found the following statistically significant results: BD patients in his study showed an increase in the amount of stage I sleep; a decrease in stage III and IV sleep; abnormal REM sleep percentages; and "a shortening of the REM latency time."[209] Gulekon et al published a report on the sleep patterns of twelve BD patients in 1993, and came to the following conclusions: the total duration of REM sleep was decreased in the majority of their BD subjects, and REM latency was increased. The researchers noted that these results are usually seen in people who are depressed; however, they had taken care to eliminate patients with psychiatric symptoms or disorders from their study. Therefore, they felt that the sleep dysfunction was caused by Behçet's, rather than depression.[210]

Treatment for disease-related fatigue can range from the use of psychostimulants or other drugs [see **Treatments** chapter later in this book] to an increase in physical activity.

Can Behçet's cause recurring fevers?
Yes. Fever can be a common feature of Behçet's disease, and may precede a general symptom flare-up by days or weeks.[139] Some cases of long-term fever have been reported, including a 39-year-old female patient whose fever lasted for two months.[140] Recurrent fever attacks have also been described as an unusual feature of Behçet's in children.[141,142] And finally, 19% of neuro-Behçet's patients in a 1999 study

by Akman-Demir showed evidence of fever during a flare-up, or specific episodes of high fever.[138]

What about unusually _low_ body temperatures?
Some Behçet's patients have personally described lower-than-normal measurable body temperatures prior to or during a symptom flare-up, although only one mention of this phenomenon was found in the literature - a brief reference to "decreased _or_ elevated temperature" prior to an acute BD attack.[139]

I seem to have more cavities than anyone I know. Can Behçet's cause cavities?
Other than Celenligil-Nazliel's mention of a 1972 study by Aoki and Choo,[159] there is little discussion in the literature of any direct link between Behçet's disease and an increase in cavities. (Aoki's study also demonstrated a higher incidence of tonsillitis in BD patients). However, one study was found that investigated the general incidence of cavities in patients with rheumatic disease. Zivkovic et al (1989) discovered that more cavities, and a higher number of extracted teeth, were found in rheumatic disease patients who were treated with corticosteroids, than in patients treated with NSAIDS or standard analgesics.[203]

Kaneko (1997) feels that Behçet's patients have an increased susceptibility to developing cavities, due to the patients' general hyper-immune response to infections.[38] Celenligil-Nazliel et al also feel that continual episodes of mouth ulcerations can prevent patients from using good oral hygiene - in other words, it hurts too much to brush and floss, so there is a higher plaque build-up and greater potential for cavity development. In 1999, Celenligil-Nazliel performed dental exams on 33 patients with Behçet's disease, and on 15 healthy subjects. Eighteen of the patients had active BD symptoms, and 15 patients were "quiet." The researchers found that there were significantly higher plaque levels in the patients with active disease, as well as higher amounts of gum inflammation and sulcular bleeding [the sulculus is the space between the tooth surface and the gums]. Probing depth [examining for gingival "pockets"] also showed higher scores in the BD patients. The number of cavities was not recorded. Curiously, there was no difference found in the total number of remaining teeth, between the patients and the healthy control subjects.

In addition to Celenligil-Nazliel's research, several studies have looked at the effect that dental work can have on the future health of patients. Kaneko found that Behçet's-related symptom flare-ups can occur following dental treatment,[38] and may be caused by over-reaction to streptococci. The antibiotic minocycline may reduce the frequency and amount of these flares. In 1988, Mizushima reported on six Behçet's patients, two of whom had severe symptom flares following dental work, and four other patients who had similar Behçet's-type symptoms following a streptococcal antigen skin test.[41] Suga (1995) reported on a Behçet's patient whose gums and cavity-filled teeth were infected with methicillin-resistant Staphylococcus aureus. The infection also caused a general flare-up of Behçet's symptoms, with severe ulcers in the mouth, and on the genitals and legs. The patient recovered after extraction of the infected teeth, and treatment with systemic vancomycin hydrochloride.[39] *[Additional information on cavities can be found on page 20, under "dry mouth."]*

I never seem to hear what people say when they talk to me anymore, and my family keeps telling me to get my hearing checked. My doctor says my ears are fine and a certain amount of hearing loss can happen as people get older. Now what?
As people age, their ability to hear high-pitched tones may diminish, whether or not they have Behcet's. Since some consonant sounds (for example, k, t, s, p and ch) contain high-pitched tones, hearing these sounds may be difficult. This can make it seem as if people around you are mumbling, or not speaking clearly.[43] However, research has shown that Behçet's disease can also affect the hearing of anywhere from 12-80% of patients. Soylu et al (1995) did a review of previous studies, and conducted their own research with 72 BD patients.[44] They found that 20 (27%) of their BD patients showed some amount of hearing loss, although not all of the patients were aware of it. (Twenty-one percent had abnormal audiograms, but had no complaints about their hearing. Only 7% complained of hearing loss, and *also* had abnormal test results.) Significant hearing losses were recorded at four specific frequencies: 0.25, 0.5, 2, and 4 kHz. There was no significant relationship found between hearing loss and any other Behçet's symptoms, or between hearing loss and the length of time that the patients had BD - although older patients tended to be the ones with more hearing-related problems. Hearing loss was one-sided in thirteen of the patients, and occurred in both ears of the other seven. According to Evereklioglu et al, "hearing loss occurs more often in older patients, and also in the complete form of Behçet's syndrome."[187] The researchers also feel that audio-vestibular involvement is underestimated in BD patients, and that patients should have regular follow-up exams by an otolaryngologist.

Other studies have shown that Behçet's can involve lesions or inflammation of the inner ear, with vestibular and/or cochlear problems;[45,46,47,48] these internal lesions may be present despite normal external ear (otoscopic) exams.[187] Dizziness, tinnitus, sudden deafness, nystagmus [constant, involuntary eyeball movements] or a feeling of pressure in the ears can be a result of involvement of the inner ear. Gemignani et al (1991) states that sudden [temporary] deafness can be a first sign of BD-related hearing problems, and that vestibular lesions can be an early sign of neuro-Behçet's. He also feels that oto-neurological testing can find hidden brainstem lesions in Behçet's patients - even in patients who have no obvious neurological problems at the time.[49] Narvaez (1998) proposes that BD-related hearing impairment should be

treated quickly, to prevent permanent hearing loss.[50] Treatment suggestions include high-dose cortisone, immunosuppressive drugs, pulse-
dose methylprednisolone, high-dose IV cyclophosphamide, and cyclosporine A.[46,50,51,52,233] Topamax was suggested to me by an RN who is also
a BD patient.

According to Szilvassy et al, if necessary it is possible to perform a cochlear implant in a patient with Behçet's disease. *[JZ: Interested readers can search out* **Cochlear implantation of a Hungar-
ian deaf and blind patient with discharging ears suffering
from Behçet's disease**, *J Laryngol Otol 1998 Feb;112(2):169-71].*

**Sometimes I feel really dizzy and have to hold on to the furni-
ture for support. After a couple of minutes I feel ok again.
Should I see my doctor?**

Yes. Some kinds of dizziness can be caused by Behçet's-related complications, but dizziness can also be a sign of other medical problems. You
can help your doctor discover the reason for your dizziness by describing in detail how you feel, since your definition of dizziness may differ
from your doctor's. For example, do you feel lightheaded, like you're
going to faint? Does dizziness happen when you stand up suddenly, or
does it occur when you're walking, or sitting, or lying down? Do you
lose your hearing temporarily, or does your vision start to fade? Do you
have a headache? Are you breathing quickly, or feeling anxious that
day? Does it feel like the room is spinning around you, or that you're
moving even though you're standing still? (This last phenomenon is
actually known as vertigo, not dizziness.) Answers to these questions can
help your doctor decide what medical tests to perform, if any.

There are many different reasons for attacks of dizziness and
vertigo. General light-headedness could be caused by anxiety, panic
attacks or other stress-related problems. Dizziness can result from low
blood pressure, from "postural changes" (standing up suddenly), from
problems in heart rhythm, or problems with the autonomic nervous
system (ANS).[53,54] However, both heart rhythm problems and ANS
complications have been known to occur in Behçet's patients.[56,57]

Vertigo (that "spinning of the room" sensation) could occur
because of lesions in the inner ear, or lesions at the eighth cranial nerve,
the brainstem, or the cerebral cortex. Inner ear, eighth cranial nerve,
and brainstem lesions can occur in Behçet's disease.[55] In some rare
cases, vertigo can also be evidence of a temporal lobe seizure.[53] If
attacks of vertigo lasting 30 minutes to 24 hours are accompanied by
fluctuating hearing loss, tinnitus and feelings of "aural fullness," then
Meniere's disease is a possibility. Treatment of Meniere's may include a
dietetic salt restriction, or the use of intratympanal gentamicin.[136]

Your doctor may refer you to a hearing specialist (ENT), a
cardiologist, or to a neurologist for further testing. Depending on your
symptoms, tests could include any of the following: an audiogram

[hearing test], EKG [electrocardiogram, which records the electrical activity of the heart], neurological exam, EEG [electroencephalogram, which records electrical activity in the brain], CT [computerized tomography or CAT scan, which uses a computer to produce cross-section pictures of the target organ(s)], or MRI [magnetic resonance imaging, which uses magnetic fields to create images of internal organs or tissues].

I've had a couple of seizures. Are they related to Behçet's?
There are many possible reasons for seizures to occur. While Behçet's studies have shown that some patients do have seizures, only your primary care physician and/or your neurologist can help to determine the exact cause.

According to the **Merck Manual of Medical Information**, a seizure is "the response to an abnormal electrical discharge in the brain," and it lasts for only a few minutes at a time. Approximately 2% of all adults will have a seizure at some point in their lives. One third of those adults will have recurrent seizures (epilepsy), while the rest will never have another episode.[110]

Depending on the part of the brain where the seizure originates, and how widely the electrical discharge spreads, symptoms may vary from mild to severe. For example: a **simple partial seizure** may result in an abnormal movement of a single muscle or limb, or the strong, unexpected sensation of a particular odor. A **febrile seizure** occurs most often as a one-time event, in a child who has a high fever. **Complex partial seizures** cause the patient to temporarily lose contact with his or her surroundings, and stare or move aimlessly. **Myoclonic seizures** are "brief, lightning-like jerks of a limb, several limbs, or the trunk."[111] In myoclonic seizures, the patient stays conscious, and these movements may or may not progress to a tonic-clonic seizure. A **tonic-clonic seizure** causes a loss of consciousness, falling, and muscle contractions in the trunk, head, arms and legs. **Status epilepticus** is a very serious situation where a seizure does not stop, and can result in the patient's death without prompt medical treatment.

Seizures can have many different causes, including brain infections (such as meningitis or viral encephalitis), metabolic problems (such as high or low levels of sugar or sodium in the blood), stroke, brain lesion(s), alcohol or drug/substance overdoses, or as an adverse reaction to some prescribed medications (such as Thorazine, Indocin or Theophylline).[110]

Behçet's patients have been known to have seizures, although according to Akman-Demir et al (1999) seizures occur in less than 5% of BD patients who have neurological involvement.[109] Six percent of the neuro-BD patients in a 1999 study by Kidd et al exhibited seizure activity. MRI results of these patients showed multiple white matter lesions in both hemispheres of the brain.[112] In 2000, a published letter by Mead, Kidd and Good described a Behçet's patient who had complex partial seizures, with an MRI that showed a medial temporal lobe lesion. The lesion disappeared within six months, following treatment with prednisolone,[113] and it was not necessary for the patient to take any anti-seizure medications. Mead, Kidd and Good provided a quick literature review at the end of their letter, and indicated several other published reports of BD patients where the following types of seizures were reported: generalized seizures, status epilepticus, and myoclonic jerks.

It's also possible for Behçet's patients to experience seizures as a result of medications taken to control their symptoms. For example, interferon alpha[115,116] and cyclosporine[121] have both been linked to seizure episodes. In addition, children with nephrotic syndrome who take chlorambucil (Leukeran) may also increase their risk of seizures.[120]

There are very few studies describing EEG test results of Behçet's patients. The patient mentioned above by Mead, Kidd and Good had a "non-specific" EEG, showing "mild asymmetry of alpha-rhythm being lower amplitude and less well-formed on the left, but no epileptiform features." However, in 1984, Matsumoto reviewed the EEGs of ten neuro-Behçet's patients. In eight cases, the EEGs showed a "mild to moderate increase in slowed alpha and theta waves, and in five cases diffuse alpha patterns. In two cases, large slow wave patterns were observed, and in Case 10, large slow waves changed into low-voltage fast dominant patterns following the status epilepticus."[114]

And finally a Behçet's patient, who had been experiencing vividly-colored, geometrically-shaped visual hallucinations at night along with feelings of dissociation, presented the following sleep-deprived EEG report from a neurologist: "This is an abnormal EEG because of the recurring sharp wave activity noted primarily in the left hemisphere, maximum in the mid-temporal central region, with some spread to the right side. The findings are consistent with a seizure disorder." A second neurologist disagreed with the report, stating that the waves were slow, rather than sharp. Regardless of the differing opinions, this patient's visual hallucinations (appearing only with the eyes closed), periodic headaches, dizziness, and peripheral neuropathy slowly resolved within six months, and a follow-up sleep-deprived EEG was normal. No anti-seizure medication was prescribed, either before or after the testing. It is interesting to note that after much research, precise descriptions of these visual hallucinations were finally found in Oliver Sacks' book, "*Migraine*;" they appeared as examples of "deep migraine aura states," the most complex of three levels of geometrical hallucinations. According to Sacks: "Some patients may observe, on closing the eyes, a form of visual tumult or delirium, in which latticed, faceted and tessellated motifs predominate - images reminiscent of mosaics, honeycombs, Turkish carpets, etc., or moiré patterns. These figments and elementary images tend to be brilliantly luminous, coloured, highly unstable, and prone to sudden kaleidoscopic transformations....there will have occurred, perhaps in the space of twenty minutes, such a revelation of bewildering (and perhaps beautiful) complexity as the mind may never be able to forget."[204] Amazingly, the patient's mind "usually remains clear...even in the stormiest migraine aura." Sacks also reported on a paper written in 1895 by Gowers, that distinguished between the electrical discharges of epileptic seizures, and those found in sensory migraine auras. Sacks' descriptions did much to explain the non-seizure nature of the geometric hallucinations described above.

Sometimes I have tremors in my hands. Are these tremors related to Behcet's disease?
Hand tremors can be caused by some medications, and/or by specific medical conditions. A neurologist is most qualified to find the cause of any tremors that you may be experiencing; however, tremors have been noted in some cases of Behçet's. In 1998 Bogdanova referred to this neuro-Behçet's complication, seen in one of his patients, as "Parkinsonian syndrome."[143] Arm and leg muscles may feel rigid, there may be a shaking of the hands and/or feet, and some jerking of tongue and facial muscles may occur. An MRI performed on Bogdanova's patient showed lesions in the substantia nigra and basal ganglia. In a 1988 review of neurological signs and symptoms of BD, Lesser and DeHoratius included tremors on a long list of previously-reported neuro-Behçet's complications.[144]

What is DVT?
DVT stands for deep vein thrombosis, which is the clotting of blood in the deep veins (located in the muscles) of the leg. The deep veins are important because they are responsible for pushing blood upward, through the legs, and back to the heart. Since there is not enough blood pressure in the leg veins to carry this blood back to the heart on its own, calf muscles help to push the blood higher with every step that a person takes, or with each time that the calf muscles are flexed. When someone is on a long trip, or put on bed rest with little movement, blood flow in the legs slows and there's an increased risk of a thrombus, or blood clot, forming in the deep veins. This can be dangerous if the thrombus breaks loose from the vein - becoming an embolus - and can be life-threatening. Approximately 20% of untreated DVTs that occur above the calf progress to a pulmonary embolism, of which 10-20% are fatal.[122]

According to the ***Merck Manual of Medical Information***, up to 50% of people with deep vein thrombosis have no symptoms; their first sign of trouble may be chest pain that indicates a pulmonary embolism. However, the following physical signs have been known to occur in patients with DVT: swelling, pain or tenderness in the calf, ankle, foot or thigh; low-grade fever; and reddish-purple, blue, or pale white discoloration of the leg.[123]

A study by Houman et al (2000) examined the records of 100 Behçet's patients in Tunisia. They found that 31% of the patients developed DVT, with men at much higher risk than women.[128] In Samangooei's study (2000), men had more vascular complications in general than women; deep vein thrombosis accounted for 39% of those vascular incidents. Samangooei also found that the presence of any one vascular problem increased the likelihood of more vascular events occurring in the same Behçet's patient.[130]

Treatment for DVT may include the use of the following drugs: anticoagulants such as heparin (Hep-Lock), warfarin (Coumadin), enoxaparin (Lovenox), tinzaparin (Innohep); or thrombolytic medications such as t-PA (Activase), urokinase (Abbokinase), or streptokinase (Kabikinase).[122]

What's wrong with my blood vessels?
The vasculitis of Behçet's can cause blood vessels of any size to become inflamed. In many cases, your symptoms can depend on the location of these inflamed blood vessels. According to Plotkin (1988) there are four specific types of problems that may occur in the blood vessels of BD patients: arterial occlusion [blocked artery]; aneurysm [abnormal dilation of a blood vessel, usually an artery, caused by a congenital problem or a weakness of the blood vessel wall]; venous occlusion [blocked vein]; and development of varices [tortuous (extremely twisted) expansions of a vein].[124] It's important to remember that not all Behçet's patients develop these vascular problems.

In a retrospective study of 1200 BD patients' records at a hospital in Turkey (Kuzu et al, 1994), there were vein complications in 14% of the patients, while approximately 2% had arterial difficulties. This total of 16% falls within Kuzu's estimate of 7-29% of BD patients who exhibit vascular problems. The specific venous problems listed in Kuzu's report included: venous thrombosis (the most common, at 13% of the cases), followed by superior vena cava syndrome, inferior vena cava syndrome, varices, upper extremity venous thrombosis, internal jugular vein thrombosis, cavernous sinus thrombosis, and hepatic vein thrombosis. Arterial problems included the following: femoral, abdominal, popliteal, iliac, pulmonary, axillary and carotid artery aneurysms, and arterial occlusions.[125]

Other researchers have reported higher frequencies of vascular lesions in their patients. For example, Sagdic et al (1996) found that 40% of BD patients in their study had vascular lesions, and that deep vein thrombosis was the most prevalent complication (in 76% of patients with vascular symptoms), followed by superficial thrombophlebitis (10%), and superior vena cava thrombosis (10%).[126] Al-Dalaan et al (2000) reported that 33% of 208 Saudi Arabian Behçet's patients in his review showed vascular problems.[129] Plotkin's 1988 estimate of the frequency of thrombophlebitis in BD patients ranged from 25-65%, depending on the study under review. In addition, he reported that thrombophlebitis can occur after minor trauma to the skin, but it can also occur spontaneously in some BD cases.[124]

Superficial thrombophlebitis is inflammation and clotting that occurs in a vein near the surface of the skin. It can cause pain, redness, and swelling, and the involved vein will feel hard to the touch. A 1992 study by Grana Gil et al found that 46% of their BD patients had vascular problems, and of that group, 92% exhibited superficial thrombophlebitis.[127] Superficial thrombophlebitis can be caused by the injury of a surface vein, through such situations as IV insertion or standard injections.

My cholesterol levels seem to have some wild swings. Is this part of Behcet's?

Some Behcet's patients do have a definite problem with how lipids [fats] are processed. Two recent studies by Orem et al (1995 and 1999) showed significant lipid-processing differences between BD patients and healthy control subjects: the BD patients' total cholesterol and LDL ("bad") cholesterol levels were increased, while triacylglycerol and HDL ("good") cholesterol levels were decreased in the same patients. Plasma lipoprotein(a) levels also varied according to the amount of disease activity.[171,172] Other studies show that the standard cholesterol indicators are not addressing the actual culprit. Erem et al (2000) found **no** differences between patients and healthy subjects in total cholesterol, LDL or HDL levels. However, as in Orem's studies, there was a significantly higher level of plasma lipoprotein(a) concentrations in the Behcet's patients, as well as a significant correlation between Lp(a) concentrations and levels of neurologic, articular, ocular and dermatologic involvement in the BD patients.[173]

Why am I losing my hair??

There are no research studies specifically linking BD to this problem, although hair loss (alopecia) can occur in other diseases such as rheumatoid arthritis, scleroderma, Crohn's, and systemic lupus erythematosus (SLE). For example, two studies in the 1990s showed that anywhere from 10-50% of SLE patients experienced hair loss that coincided with increases in the activity of their disease.[152,153]

Hair loss in Behcet's patients can be caused by many different factors, but is most likely a temporary medication side effect. Drugs that may cause a certain amount of hair loss include colchicine; azathioprine (Imuran); interferon alpha-2a; leflunomide (Arava); cyclophosphamide (Cytoxan); celecoxib (Celebrex); mesalazine (Pentasa); methotrexate (Folex); trimethadione (Tridione); beta blocker drugs such as propranolol (Inderal) for high blood pressure; and blood thinners such as Heparin.[154] If hair loss is a concern for you, please ask your health care provider how much (if any) hair loss to expect with the drugs prescribed for your care.

According to the CDC, other possible reasons for hair loss can include the following: high fevers, hormonal changes, pregnancy, surgical shock, transplant surgery, aging, male pattern baldness, poor diet, anemia, decreased thyroid levels, and severe emotional stress.[155] In addition, scarring of the scalp (as a result of infections or continual scalp lesions, for example) may make it difficult for hair to grow back normally.[156]

In the future, it may be possible for cyclin-dependent kinases (CDKs) to be used to prevent hair loss caused by chemotherapy drugs. A 2001 study by Meijer et al reported that Glaxo Wellcome unexpectedly discovered this beneficial side effect during their company's research.[157]

Can my lungs be affected by Behcet's?

Yes. Lee (2001) looked at the results of research studies from ten different countries, and found that pulmonary (lung) involvement occurred in less than 1% of the Behçet's patients examined in China and Iran, and ranged up to a high of 36% of the patients enrolled in a Greek study.[175] In a review of the literature, Papiris and Moutsopoulos (1993) found the main symptoms of respiratory involvement to be cough, hemoptysis [coughing up blood, a serious complication needing immediate attention], dyspnea [difficulty in breathing] and pleuritic chest pain [the pleura is the membrane surrounding both lungs].[176] Raz et al (1989) discovered that almost 10% of their patients had pulmonary vasculitis; most of these patients were young men, who also exhibited fever, anemia, and an elevated ESR.[177] Dilsen et al (1991) noted that six times as many men were diagnosed with BD-related lung involvement in their research than women. They also found that those patients with pulmonary problems were more likely to have eye problems, as well as amyloidosis. In addition, they saw higher amounts of thrombophlebitis in their respiratory patients.[178]

According to Plotkin's 1988 review of BD-related respiratory involvement (in ***Behçet's Disease: A Contemporary Synopsis***) it's possible for any part of the respiratory tract to be affected - from the nose down to the lungs. He states that the following problems have been noted in Behçet's patients with upper respiratory involvement: "rhinorrhea [runny nose], recurrent sore throats, tonsillitis, and dysphonia [hoarseness]."[174] Of course, these health problems may also occur as part of a normal cold or other illness; pay close attention to any additional symptoms taking place, so that your doctor can be consulted for appropriate treatment. Behçet's-related ulcerations have been found in/on the following places: the bronchi, pharynx, larynx, tonsils, palate and epiglottis [the "punching bag" at the top of the throat]. If these ulcers are severe and frequent, they may result in scar tissue or narrowed openings that cause difficulty in speaking, swallowing or breathing.[174]

For clinicians reading this section, pulmonary artery aneurysms were seen in more than half of Raz's respiratory patients in 1989. In addition, "chest x-ray films showed pulmonary infiltrates, pleural effusions [fluid in the chest cavity], and prominent pulmonary arteries.

Ventilation-perfusion scans showed perfusion defects even when chest x-ray films were normal."[177] The following imaging results have also been found (Dilsen et al, 1991): "well-defined opacities and nodular lesions, linear or other types of atelectasis, hilar enlargement, diaphragmatic elevation, ill-defined opacities, and sinus obliteration ... Pulmonary perfusion scintigraphy revealed multiple lobar segmental or multiple peripheral defects." CT scan findings included central and peripheral aneurysms, widening or narrowing of the pulmonary arteries and/or irregularities of their walls, hilar or mediastinal lymphadenopathy, and parenchymal infiltrations.[178]

Can Behçet's cause heart problems?
Yes, several studies have shown cardiac problems in BD patients. In a 1993 literature review, Schiff et al acknowledged that pericarditis, myocarditis, atrial fibrillation and conduction disturbances have been found in cases of Behçet's.[211] Their own report described a Behçet's patient who suffered a heart attack owing to blockage of a coronary artery caused by BD-related artery inflammation. In a study of 350 Egyptian patients in 1993, Assaad-Khalil et al found that 15% of their subjects demonstrated heart problems that included mitral valve prolapse, pericarditis, heart attack, asymmetrical sepal hypertrophy, or a left ventricular aneurysm.[212] Other cardiac manifestations included supraventricular arrythmias (abnormal heart rhythms), and silent myocardial ischaemia (temporary decrease in blood flow to that area, due to a circulation blockage). In 1996, Morelli et al stated that "patients with Behçet's disease show an unusually high prevalence of clinically silent cardiac abnormalities like mitral valve prolapse and aortic root dilatation."[213] Mitral valve prolapse was seen in 50% of their study subjects, and 30% displayed proximal aorta dilatation. Morelli et al suggested serial echocardiographic testing to screen for these problems. (The high incidence of mitral valve prolapse was in strong contrast to Ozkam et al's results in BD patients - only 6% of Ozkam's subjects showed MVP.) Morelli also found that there was a significant relationship between the length of time their patients had BD, and the diameter of the patients' ascending aorta.

A report by Mirone et al (1997) described a young woman who developed tachycardia (an abnormally fast heart rhythm) three years after her BD diagnosis. Her heart rhythm disturbances increased when she had BD-related symptom flares in other parts of her body.[214] Mirone concluded that the woman's arrhythmias were probably due to myocarditis (inflammation of cardiac muscle) caused by Behçet's. A study by Goldeli et al (1997) found significant increases in QT and JT dispersion values in their BD patients with ventricular arrhythmias, and suggested that the test be used as a diagnostic tool.[215]

In 2001, Tellioglu and Robertson described a case of orthostatic intolerance in a Behçet's patient. Orthostatic intolerance causes a variety of symptoms upon standing: a fast heart rate, lightheadedness, fatigue, altered thinking patterns, and/or fainting spells. The researchers' 19-year-old subject found that when she stood up, her pulse rate shot into the 160s, and her blood pressure fell to 80/40, causing fainting spells. According to Tellioglu and Robertson, "this is the first [published study] to suggest the pathophysiology of BD as a potential cause of autonomic dysregulation resulting in OI [orthostatic intolerance]."[234]

There are times when my heart suddenly starts beating fast, and I feel dizzy, anxious, and short of breath. My doctor says I'm having a panic attack, but I'm not upset or overly concerned about my life or my relationships. What's going on? According to *Taber's Cyclopedic Medical Dictionary*, a panic attack is "acute intense anxiety; symptoms include dyspnea (trouble breathing), sweating, vertigo, palpitations, chest pain, nausea, blurred vision, dread, feeling that there will be loss of mental control, and feeling of approaching death." If you have questions about how (or if) these symptoms relate to your emotional health, you should speak in depth with your primary care physician. You may be given a referral to a mental health professional for additional follow-up, and/or be given a prescription for medicine to help decrease or eliminate these attacks.

It is also possible that the above symptoms are instead caused by medications, or by a problem with your autonomic nervous system due to "sympathetic hyperreactivity" from Behçet's.[216] A 1991 study by Dilsen et al found the following symptoms in BD patients, and concluded that they indicated an increase in the activity of the sympathetic nervous system, compared with healthy control subjects: "hyperperspiration of hands and body, supersensitivity to stress, cramps in legs, muscular pain, and sweating with [hot] flashes." The sympathetic nervous system is part of the autonomic nervous system; it helps with the "fight or flight" response that gets the body ready for emergency or otherwise-stressful situations. Aksyek et al agreed with Dilsen in 1999, by stating that "patients with Behçet's disease may have asymptomatic ANS dysfunction, which is in the form of increased sympathetic... modulation."[217] They suggest that power spectral analysis of heart rate variability can help to evaluate the autonomic nervous system in BD patients.

As we saw in the question about fatigue and sleep earlier in this chapter, the autonomic nervous system regulates heart and breathing rates, blood pressure, body tempreature, and other functions that operate without conscious effort--in essence, some of the same functions that are also disrupted during a panic attack. It may be no coincidence that the brainstem plays a part in regulation of the autonomic nervous system-- and that the brain stem is also a primary location for Behcet's lesions.

References

(1) Lee, Bang, Lee and Sohn (Eds). Behçet's Disease: A Guide to its Clinical Understanding. Springer Verlag, Berlin, c2001, p 13

(2) Estimation of case numbers based on 2000 population figures supplied by the Population Reference Bureau @ www.prb.org, 5/01.

(3) Zeis, J (2001) Basic information on Behçet's disease, p 6.

(4) Teter MS, Hochberg MC (1988) Diagnostic criteria and epidemiology. In: Plotkin GR, Calabro JJ, O'Duffy JD (eds) Behçet's Disease: a Contemporary Synopsis. Futura Publishing Co., New York, p 16.

(5) Lee S et al (2001) Behçet's Disease: A Guide to its Clinical Understanding. Springer Verlag, Berlin, p 1.

(6) Friedman-Birdbaum et al. Sensitivity and specificity of pathergy test results in Israeli patients with Behçet's disease. Cutis 1990 45:261-264

(7) Davies PG, Fordham JN, Kirwan JR, Barnes CG, Dinning WJ. The pathergy test and Behcet's syndrome in Britain. Ann Rheum Dis 1984 Feb;43(1):70-3.

(8) Fresko I, Yazici H, Bayramicli M, Yurdakul S, Mat C. Effect of surgical cleaning of the skin on the pathergy phenomenon in Behçet's syndrome. Ann Rheum Dis 1993 Aug;52(8):619-20

(9) Dilsen N, Konice M, Aral O, Ocal L, Inanc M, Gul A. Comparative study of the skin pathergy test with blunt and sharp needles in Behçet's disease: confirmed specificity but decreased sensitivity with sharp needles. Ann Rheum Dis 1993 Nov;52(11):823-5

(10) Ozarmagan G, Saylan T et al. Re-evaluation of the pathergy test in Behçet's disease; 1991 71(1):75-6

(11) Lee S et al (2001) Behçet's Disease: A Guide to its Clinical Understanding. Springer Verlag, Berlin, p 17

(12) O'Duffy JD et al. HLA antigens in Behçet's disease. J Rheumatol 1976 3:1-3

(13) Yazici H et al. HLA antigens in Behçet's disease: a reappraisal by a comparative study of Turkish and British patients. Ann Rheum Dis 1980 39:344-348

(14) Verity DH et al. Behçet's disease, the Silk Road and HLA-B51: historical and geographical perspectives. Tissue Antigens. 1999 Sep;54(3):213-20

(15) Yabuki K et al. Association of MICA gene and HLA-B*5101 with Behçet's disease in Greece. Invest Ophthalmol Vis Sci. 1999 Aug;40(9):1921-6

(16) Mizuki N et al. Triplet repeat polymorphism in the transmembrane region of the MICA gene: a strong association of six GCT repetitions with Behcet disease. Proc Natl Acad Sci U S A. 1997 Feb 18;94(4):1298-303

(17) Orloff LA, Orloff MJ. Budd-Chiari syndrome caused by Behçet's disease: treatment by side-to-side portacaval shunt; J Am Coll Surg 1999 Apr;188(4):396-407

(18) Yazici H et al. The ten-year mortality in Behçet's sydrome. Br J Rheumatol 1996 Feb;35(2):139-41

(19) Park KD, Bang D, Lee ES, Lee SH, Lee S. Clinical study on death in Behçet's disease. J Korean Med Sci 1993 Aug;8(4):241-5

(20) Walsh SJ, Rau LM. Autoimmune diseases: a leading cause of death among young and middle-aged women in the United States. Am J Public Health 2000 Sep;90(9):1463-6

(21) Plotkin G (1988). Miscellaneous clinical manifestations: renal complications. In: Plotkin GR, Calabro JJ, O'Duffy JD (eds) Behçet's disease: a contemporary synopsis. Futura Publishing Co, New York, pp 214-20

(22) Pickering, MC. False-positive results obtained using the Mantoux test in Behçet's syndrome: comment on the article by Garcia-Porrua et al. Arthritis Rheum 2000 Dec;43(12):2855-6

(23) Erdogru T et al. Evaluation and therapeutic approaches of voiding and erectile dysfunction in neurological Behçet's syndrome. J Urol 1999 July;162:147-153

(24) Cetinel B et al. Bladder involvement in Behçet's syndrome. J Urol 1999 Jan;161(1):52-6

(25) Lida S et al. A case of neurogenic bladder due to neuro-Behcet disease. Hinyokika Kiyo 2000 Oct;46(10):727-9

(26) Aksu K et al. Erectile dysfunction in Behçet's disease without neurological

involvement: two case reports. Rheumatology 2000;39:1429-1431

(27) Scheid P, Bohadana A, Martinet Y. Nicotine patches for aphthous ulcers due to Behçet's syndrome. NEJM 2000 Dec 14(343);24:1816-7

(28) Baron JA. Beneficial effects of nicotine and cigarette smoking: the real, the possible and the spurious. Br Med Bull 1996 Jan;52(1):58-73

(29) Bittoun R. Recurrent aphthous ulcers and nicotine. Med J Aust 1991 Apr 1;154(7):471-2

(30) Grady D et al. Smokeless tobacco use prevents aphthous stomatitis. Oral Surg Oral Med Oral Path 1992 Oct;74(4):463-5

(31) Krause I et al. Seasons of the year and activity of SLE and Behçet's disease. Scand J Rheumatol 1997;26(6):435-9

(32) Zatorska B et al. The seasonal course of recurrent uveitis in children and youth. Klin Oczna 2000;102(4):263-6

(33) Schaefer KM. Health patterns of women with fibromyalgia. J Adv Nurs 1997 Sep;26(3):565-71

(34) Affleck G. Attributional processes in rheumatoid arthritis patients. Arthritis Rheum 1987 Aug;30(8):927-31

(35) White AT et al. Effect of precooling on physical performance in multiple sclerosis. Mult Scler 2000 Jun;6(3):176-80

(36) Hawley DJ, Wolfe F, Lue FA, Moldofsky H. Seasonal symptom severity in patients with rheumatic diseases: a study of 1,424 patients. J Rheumatol 2001 Aug;28(8):1900-9

(37) Bang D et al. Epidemiological and clinical features of Behçet's disease in Korea. Appendix 13 in Lee, Bang, Lee and Sohn (eds), Behçet's Disease: A Guide to its Clinical Understanding. Copyright 2001 Springer-Verlag, Germany

(38) Kaneko F, Oyama N, Nishibu A. Streptococcal infection in the pathogenesis of Behçet's disease and clinical effects of minocycline on the disease symptoms. Yonsei Med J 1997 Dec;38(6):444-54

(39) Suga Y et al. A case of Behçet's disease aggravated by gingival infection with methicillin-resistant Staphylococcus aureus. Br J Dermatol 1995 Aug;133(2):319-21

(40) Lee S et al. A study of HLA antigens in Behçet's syndrome. Yonsei Med J 1988;29:259-262

(41) Mizushima Y et al. Induction of Behçet's disease symptoms after dental treatment and streptococcal antigen skin test. J Rheumatol 1988 Jun;15(6):1029-30

(42) Axell T, Henricsson V. Association between recurrent aphthous ulcers and tobacco habits. Scand J Dent Res 1985 Jun;93(3):239-42

(43) Berkow, R (ed). The Merck Manual of Medical Information, Home Edition. Pub by Merck Research Laboratories, NJ, c. 1997;p.13

(44) Soylu L et al. Hearing loss in Behçet's disease. Ann Otol Rhinol Laryngol 1995;104:864-7

(45) Igarashi Y et al. A case of Behçet's disease with otologic symptoms. ORL J Otorhinolaryngol Relat Spec 1994 Sept-Oct;56(5):295-8

(46) Tsunoda I et al. Acute simultaneous bilateral vestibulocochlear impairment in neuro-Behçet's disease: a case report. Auris Nasus Larynx 1994;21(4):243-7

(47) Schwanitz HJ, Knop J, Bonsmann G. Behcet disease with inner ear involvement. Z Hautkr 1984 Sep 1;59(17):1173-4

(48) Belkahia A et al. Auditory and vestibular lesions in Behçet's disease. Ann Otolaryngol Chir Cervicofac 1982;99(10-11):469-76

(49) Gemignani G et al. Hearing and vestibular disturbances in Behçet's syndrome. Ann Otol Rhinol Laryngol 1991 Jun;100(6):459-63

(50) Narvaez J et al. Sudden cochlear hearing loss in a patient with Behçet's disease. Rev Rhum Engl Ed 1998 Jan;65(1):63-4

(51) Elidan J, Levi H, Cohen E, BenEzra D. Effect of cyclosporine A on the hearing loss in Behçet's disease. Ann Otol Rhinol Laryngol 1991 Jun;100(6):464-8

(52) Berrettini S et al. Sudden deafness and Behçet's disease. Acta otorhinolaryngol Belg 1989;43(3):221-9

(53) Duman S, Ginsburg S. "Dizziness and Vertigo" in Problem-Oriented Medical

Diagnosis, 6th Ed. (Friedman, H ed); 1996, Little,Brown & Co, Boston. pp 410-3
(54) Martin G (ed). "Dizziness (Causes/Approach/Treatment Options)" in
Consumer Guide's Your Family's Guide to Symptoms and Treatments. 1997,
Publications International, pp 36-9
(55) Kidd D, Steuer A, Denman AM, Rudge P. Neurological complications in
Behçet's syndrome. Brain 1999;122:2183-94
(56) Aksovek S et al. Assessment of autonomic nervous system function in patients
with Behcet's disease by spectral analysis of heart rate variability. J Auton Nerv
Syst. 1999 Sep 24;77(2-3): 190-4
(57) Kirimli O et al. Heart rate variability, late potentials and QT dispersion as
markers of myocardial involvement in patients with Behçet's disease. Can J
Cardiol. 2000 Mar;16(3):345-51
(58) Berkow, R (ed). The Merck Manual of Medical Information, Home Edition.
Pub by Merck Research Laboratories, NJ, c. 1997;p.1065
(59) Kaklamani VG, Kaklamanis PG. Treatment of Behçet's disease: an update.
Semin Arthritis Rheum 2001 Apr;30(5):299-312
(60) Berkow, R (ed). The Merck Manual of Medical Information, Home Edition.
Pub by Merck Research Laboratories, NJ, c. 1997;p.632
(61) Azizlerli G et al. A new kind of skin lesion in Behçet's disease: extragenital
ulcerations. Acta Derm Venereol 1992 Aug;72(4):286
(62) Chen KR, Kawahara Y, Miyakawa S, Nishikawa T. Cutaneous vasculitis in
Behçet's disease: a clinical and histopathologic study of 20 patients. J Am Acad
Dermatol 1997 May;36(5 Pt 1): 689-96
(63) Plotkin G (1988). Triple Symptom Complex: Genital Ulcers. In: Plotkin GR,
Calabro JJ, O'Duffy JD (eds) Behçet's Disease: A Contemporary Synopsis. Futura
Publishing Co, New York, p 158
(64) Plotkin G (1988). Miscellaneous Clinical Manifestations, II: Dermatologic
Manifestations. In: Plotkin GR, Calabro JJ, O'Duffy JD (eds) Behçet's Disease: A
Contemporary Synopsis. Futura Publishing Co, New York, p 258
(65) Ship JA et al. Recurrent aphthous stomatitis. Quintessence International
2000;31(2):95-108.
(66) Lakhanpal S, O'Duffy JD and Lie JT. Ophthalmic Pathology. In: Behçet's
Disease: A Contemporary Synopsis. Plotkin GR, Calabro JJ, O'Duffy JD (eds)
Futura Publishing Co, New York, p130
(67) Plotkin G (1988). Uveitis. In: Behçet's Disease: A Contemporary Synopsis.
Plotkin GR, Calabro JJ, O'Duffy JD (eds), Futura Publishing Co, New York, p164
(68) Kim HB. Ophthalmologic manifestation of Behçet's disease. Yonsei Med J
1997 Dec;38(6):390-4
(69) Al-Saleh S et al. Causes of death in Behçet's disease. Yonsei Med J, 2000; 41:3
(Suppl), p50
(70) Zouboulis C. Genitoanal lesions in Adamantiades-Behcet's disease. Yonsei
Med J, 2000;41:3 (Suppl), p16
(71) Wechsler B et al. International criteria for classification of Behcet's disease. In
Behcet's Disease: Basic and Clinical Aspects. O'Duffy JD, Kokmen E (eds.), Marcel
Dekker, c1991, p33
(72) Cho MY et al. Clinical analysis of 57 cases of Behçet's syndrome in children. In
Behcet's Disease: Basic and Clinical Aspects. O'Duffy JD, Kokmen E (eds.), Marcel
Dekker, c1991, p45
(73) Russell AJ, Lawson WA and Haskard DO. Potential new therapeutic options
in Behçet's syndrome. BioDrugs 2001:15(1):25-35
(74) Sharquie K et al. Behçet's disease in Iraqi patients. A prospective study from a
newly established Behçet's Disease Multidiscipline Clinic. Yonsei Med J
2000;41(3) Suppl., p 10
(75) Madanat W et al. Influence of sex on Behçet's disease in Jordan. Yonsei Med J
2000;41(3) Suppl., p 31
(76) Cakir N, Yazici H, Chamberlain MA, et al. Response to intradermal injection of
monosodium urate crystals in Behçet's syndrome. Ann Rheum Dis 1991;50:634-6
(77) Mizuki N et al. Association analysis between the MIC-A and HLA-B alleles

in Japanese patients with Behçet's disease. Arthritis Rheum 1999;42:1961-6
(78) Mizuki N et al. Microsatellite mapping of a susceptible locus within the HLA region for Behcet's disease using Jordanian patients. Hum Immunol. 2001 Feb;62(2):186-90
(79) Salvarani C et al. Association of MICA alleles and HLA-B51 in Italian patients with Behcet's disease. J Rheumatol. 2001 Aug;28(8):1867-70
(80) Russell AI, Lawson WA and Haskard DO. Potential new therapeutic options in Behçet's syndrome. BioDrugs 2001:15(1):25-35
(81) Bang D, Kim H, Lee E, and Lee S. The significance of laboratory tests in evaluating the clinical activity of Behçet's disease. Yonsei Med J 2000;41(3) Suppl., p32
(82) Lee S and Bang D. Behcet disease. eMedicine Journal, July 2001:2(7), section 5
(83) Lee, Bang, Lee and Sohn (eds), Behçet's Disease: A Guide to its Clinical Understanding. Copyright 2001 Springer-Verlag, Germany, p55
(84) Marshall, Goman and Marciniak. (1988). Hematologic aspects. In: Behçet's Disease: A Contemporary Synopsis. Plotkin GR, Calabro JJ, O'Duffy JD (eds), Futura Publishing Co, New York, p86
(85) Lee, Bang, Lee and Sohn (eds), Behçet's Disease: A Guide to its Clinical Understanding. Copyright 2001 Springer-Verlag, Germany, p62
(86) Zouboulis CC et al. Adamantiades-Behçet's disease: interleukin-8 is increased in serum of patients with active oral and neurological manifestations and is secreted by small vessel endothelial cells. Arch Dermatol Res 2000 Jun;292(6):279-84
(87) Shaquie K, Al-Araji A, and Hatem A. Oral pathergy test. Yonsei Med J 2000;41(3)Suppl, p41
(88) Lee, Bang, Lee and Sohn (eds), Behçet's Disease: A Guide to its Clinical Understanding. Copyright 2001 Springer-Verlag, Germany, p55
(89) Ghaderi A, Samangooei Sh et al. Positive rheumatoid factor test by ELISA method in Behçet's disease. Yonsei Med J 2000;41(3) Suppl., p46
(90) Salvi F et al. Optic neuropathy in Behcet's disease. Report of two cases. Ital J Neurol Sci. 1999 Jun;20(3):183-6
(91) Kansu T et al. Optic neuropathy in Behcet's disease. J Clin Neuroophthalmol 1989 Dec;9(4):277-80
(92) Kansu T et al. Optic nerve involvement in Behçet's disease. In: Behçet's Disease: Basic and Clinical Aspects. O'Duffy JD and Kokmen E (eds), Copyright 1991 by Marcel Dekker, Inc., NY; p77-83
(93) BenEzra D. The ocular viewpoint of Behçet's disease. In: Behçet's Disease: Basic and Clinical Aspects. O'Duffy JD and Kokmen E (eds), Copyright 1991 by Marcel Dekker, Inc., NY; p93-97
(94) Plotkin GR. Uveitis (triple symptom complex). In: Behçet's Disease: A Contemporary Synopsis. Plotkin GR, Calabro JJ, O'Duffy JD (eds), Futura Publishing Co, New York, c1988, p161
(95) Pivetti-Pezzi P, Bozzoni F et al. Does unilateral ocular involvement exist in patients with Behçet's disease? Yonsei Med J 2000;41(3)Suppl, p46
(96) el Belhadji M, Hamdani M et al. [Ophthalmological involvement in Behcet disease. Apropos of 520 cases]. J Fr Ophtalmol 1997;20(8):592-8
(97) Chee, SP. Retinal vasculitis associated with systemic disease. In "Ophthalmology Clinics of North America", Stamper RL (ed);December 1998:11(4), p657-667
(98) Lakhanpal S, O'Duffy JD, Lie JT. Pathology (Cutaneous Lesions). In: Behçet's Disease: A Contemporary Synopsis. Plotkin GR, Calabro JJ, O'Duffy JD (eds), Futura Publishing Co, New York, p104
(99) Dilsen N. Risk factors in Behçet's disease. Yonsei Med J 2000;41(3)Suppl, p26
(100) Plotkin GR. Triple Symptom Complex (Genital Ulcers). In: Behçet's Disease: A Contemporary Synopsis. Plotkin GR, Calabro JJ, O'Duffy JD (eds), Futura Publishing Co, New York, p159
(101) Rogers RS 3rd. Recurrent aphthous stomatitis: clinical characteristics and associated systemic disorders. Semin Cutan Med Surg. 1997 Dec;16(4):278-83
(102) Bang D, Chun YS et al. The influence of pregnancy on Behçet's Disease;

Yonsei Med J Dec 1997;38(6):437-43

(103) Ostensen M, Rugelsjoen A, Wigers SH. The effect of reproductive events and alterations of sex hormone levels on the symptoms of fibromyalgia. Scand J Rheumatol 1997;26(5):355-60

(104) Lee S et al. Behçet's disease or Behçet's syndrome. Yonsei Med J 2000;41(3)Suppl, p9, and full presentation through personal correspondence w/ Dr. Lee, 10/01

(105) Fresko I et al. The response to the intradermal injection to monosodium urate in Behçet's syndrome (BS) and its comparison to the pathergy test. Yonsei Med J 2000;41(3) Suppl, p29

(106) Melikoglu M et al. A reappraisal of amyloidosis in Behçet's syndrome (BS). Yonsei Med J 2000;41(3)Suppl, p26

(107) Wilbur DC, Maurer S and Smith NJ. Behçet's disease in a vaginal smear. Acta Cytol 1993 Jul-Aug;37(4):525-30

(108) Aygunduz M, et al. Serum amyloid A and beta-2 microglobulin as markers of clinical activity in Behçet's disease. Yonsei Med J 2000;41(3) Suppl, p35

(109) Akman-Demir G et al. Clinical patterns of neurological involvement in Behçet's disease: evaluation of 200 patients. Brain (1999),122, 2171-2181

(110) "Seizure Disorders" in The Merck Manual of Medical Information, Home Edition. 1997, Merck & Co, NJ, 345-50

(111) "Seizure Disorders" in The Merck Manual of Diagnosis and Therapy, 17th Ed, 1999, p1401-1409

(112) Kidd D et al. Neurological complications in Behçet's syndrome. Brain(1999),122,2183-2194

(113) Mead S, Kidd D and Good C. Behçet's syndrome may present with partial seizures. J Neurol Neurosurg Psychiatry 2000;68:392-393(March)

(114) Matsumoto K. Correlation between EEG and clinicopathological change in neuro-Behçet's syndrome. Folia Psychiatr Neurol Jpn 1984;38(1):65-79

(115) O'Duffy JD et al. Interferon-alpha treatment of Behcet's disease. J Rheumatol. 1998 Oct;25(10):1938-44

(116) Ameen M, Russell-Jones R. Seizures associated with interferon-alpha treatment of cutaneous malignancies. Br J Dermatol. 1999 Aug;141(2):386-7

(117) O'Duffy JD. "Pathology and Immunopathogenesis" in Behçet's Disease. In Primer on the Rheumatic Diseases, Ed 11, 1997 Arthritis Foundation, GA, p308

(118) Kwak YT, Chang BC and Cho BK. Surgical experience of Behçet's disease involving cardiovascular system. Yonsei Med J 2000;41(3) Suppl, p19

(119) Lee CW, Lee J, et al. Aortic valve involvement in Behçet's disease. Yonsei Med J 2000;41(3) Suppl, p43

(120) PDR Nurse's Drug Handbook, c2002 Medical Economics Co, NJ. p380

(121) PDR Nurse's Drug Handbook, c2002 Medical Economics Co, NJ. P461

(122) Schreiber D. Deep venous thrombosis and thrombophlebitis. eMedicine J, October 9 2001, 2:10

(123) "Venous and Lymphatic Disorders" in The Merck Manual of Medical Information, Home Edition. 1997, Merck & Co, NJ, 141-43

(124) Plotkin G. "Miscellaneous Clinical Manifestations, Part I: Cardiac, Vascular, Renal, and Pulmonary Features" in Behçet's Disease: A Contemporary Synopsis. Plotkin G, Calabro J and O'Duffy JD (eds), c1988 Futura Publishing, NY; p207-213

(125) Kuzu MA et al. Vascular involvement in Behçet's disease: 8-year audit. World J Surg 1994 Nov-Dec;18(6):948-54

(126) Sagdic K et al. Venous lesions in Behçet's disease. Eur J Vasc Endovasc Surg 1996 May;11(4):437-40

(127) Grana Gil J et al. [Vascular manifestations in 30 cases of Behçet's disease.] [Spanish]. Rev Clin Esp 1992 Nov;191(7):375-9

(128) Houman MH et al. Deep vein thrombosis in Behçet's disease. Yonsei Med J 2000;41(3) Suppl,p44

(129) Al-Dalaan A, Al-Shaikh A, Al-Saleh S and Al-Ballaa S. Vascular manifestations of Behçet's disease. Yonsei Med J 2000;41(3) Suppl,p18

(130) Samangooei S et al. Vascular complications in 343 patients with Behçet's

disease from Shiraz, south-west of Iran. Yonsei Med J 2000;41(3) Suppl,p19

(131) Oh BH, Lee HS, Lee HL, Bang D, Lee S. Psychiatric aspects of Behçet's syndrome. Neuropsychiatry 1985;24:508-551

(132) Bhakta BB et al. Behçet's disease: evaluation of a new instrument to measure clinical activity. Rheumatology 1999;38:728-733

(133) "Rehabilitation of Patients with Rheumatic Disease" in Primer on the Rheumatic Diseases, 11th Ed, c1997 Arthritis Foundation, p410

(134) Swain MG. Fatigue in chronic disease. Clin Sci (Colch) 2000 Jul;99(1):1-8

(135) Wolfe F, Hawley DJ, Wilson K. The prevalence and meaning of fatigue in rheumatic disease. J Rheumatol 1996 Aug;23(8):1407-17

(136) Jensen JM. "Vertigo and Dizziness" in Neurology for the Non-Neurologist, Weiner WJ and Goetz CG (eds). C1999, Lippincott Williams & Wilkins, p209-210

(137) Kocer N et al. CNS involvement in neuro-Behcet syndrome: an MR study. Amer J Neuroradiology 1999;20:1015-1024

(138) Akman-Demir G, Serdaroglu P, Tasci B and the neuro-Behcet Study Group. Clinical patterns of neurological involvement in Behçet's disease: evaluation of 200 patients. Brain (1999), 122, 2171-2181

(139) Plotkin GR. "Triple Symptom Complex" in Behçet's Disease: A Contemporary Synopsis. c1999 Futura Publishing, NY, p144

(140) Granel B et al. [An unusual cause of long-term fever: Behcet disease]. Presse Med 1999 Dec 18-25;28(40):2221-2

(141) Kone-Paut I. [Behçet's disease: pediatric features]. Ann Med Interne (Paris) 1999 Nov;150(7):571-5

(142) Majeed HA. Differential diagnosis of fever of unknown origin in children. Curr Opin Rheumatol 2000 Sept;12(5):439-44

(143) Bogdanova D, Milanov I, Georgiev D. Parkinsonian syndrome as a neurological manifestation of Behçet's disease. Can J Neurol Sci 1998 Feb;25(1):82-5

(144) Lesser RS and DeHoratius RJ. "Miscellaneous Clinical Manifestations, Part III (Neuro-Behçet's Syndrome) in Behçet's Disease: A Contemporary Synopsis. c1999 Futura Publishing, NY, p283

(145) Wechsler B, Du LT, Kieffer E. [Cardiovascular manifestations of Behçet's disease]. Ann Med Interne (Paris) 1999 Nov;150(7):542-54

(146) Zouboulis CC. Epidemiology of Adamantiades-Behçet's disease. Ann Med Interne (Paris) 1999 Oct;150(6):488-98

(147) Saito M, Miyagawa I. Bladder dysfunction due to Behcet's disease.Urol Int.2000;65(1):40-2

(148) Ek L, Hedfors E. Behcet's disease: a review and a report of 12 cases from Sweden. Acta Derm Venereol. 1993 Aug;73(4):251-4

(149) Kirkali et al. Urological aspects of Behcet's disease. Br J Urol. 1991 Jun;67(6):638-9

(150) O'Duffy JD. "History and Evolution" in Behçet's Disease: A Contemporary Synopsis. Plotkin G, Calabro J and O'Duffy JD (eds), c1988 Futura Publishing, NY; p3

(151) Foster CS. Presentation at American Behçet's Disease Association Patient/ Family Conference; October 2001, Boston, MA.

(152) Wysenbeek AJ, Leibovici L, Amit M, Weinberger A. Alopecia in systemic lupus erythematosus. Relation to disease manifestations. J Rheumatol 1991 Aug;18(8):1185-6

(153) Werth VP, White WL, Sanchez MR, Franks AG. Incidence of alopecia areata in lupus erythematosus. Arch Derrmatol 1991 Mar;128(3):368-71

(154) "Common drugs that cause hair loss" in Hair Loss and Its Causes. http:// familydoctor.org/handouts/081.html

(155) "Hair loss" at http://www.cdc.gov/nip/vacsafe/concerns/Hairloss.htm, Center for Disease Control, US, 2001

(156) Hair Loss and Its Causes. http://familydoctor.org/handouts/081.html, 2001

(157) Meijer L, Knockaert M, Damiens E. [Prevention of chemotherapy-induced alopecia by cyclin-dependent kinase inhibitors]. Bull Cancer 2001 Apr;88(4):347-50

(158) Ship JA et al. Recurrent aphthous stomatitis. Quintessence Int 2000;31:95-112

(159) Celenligil-Nazliel H, Kansu E and Ebersole J. Periodontal findings and systemic antibody responses to oral microorganisms in Behçet's disease. J Periodontol 1999 December; 70(12):1449-1456
(160) Arthritis Foundation, GA. c.1999, Sjogren's syndrome brochure
(161) Arthritis Foundation, GA, c.2000, Raynaud's phenomenon brochure
(162) Alballa SR et al. HLA-B5(51) in Behçet's disease: lack of correlation with severity. In "Behçet's Disease", Godeau and Wechsler (eds), c.1993 Elsevier Science Publishers, p619-22
(163) Bodmer JG, Bodmer WF and Marsh SGE. HLA nomenclature: the name of the rose. In "HLA in Health and Disease (2nd Ed)", Lechler and Warrens (Eds.) Academic Press (2000), p149
(164) Kural E et al. The 20-year prognosis of Behçet's syndrome. Abstract from the American College of Rheumatology Conference, Philadephia, November 2000; courtesy K Calamia, MD
(165) Wechsler B et al. International criteria for classification of Behcet's disease. In Behcet's Disease: Basic and Clinical Aspects. O'Duffy JD, Kokmen E (eds.), Marcel Dekker, c1991, p32
(166) Wechsler B et al. International criteria for classification of Behcet's disease. In Behcet's Disease: Basic and Clinical Aspects. O'Duffy JD, Kokmen E (eds.), Marcel Dekker, c1991, p33
(167) Lee S et al (2001) Behçet's Disease: A Guide to its Clinical Understanding. Springer Verlag, Berlin, p52-53
(168) Chang HK, Kim JU, Cheon KS et al. HLA-B51 and its allelic types in association with Behçet's disease and recurrent aphthous stomatitis in Korea. Clin Exp Rheum 2001;19(Suppl 24):S31-S35
(169) Kaklamani VG, Nikolopoulou N, Sotsiou F, Billis A, Kaklamanis P. Renal involvement in Adamantiades-Behçet's disease. Case report and review of the literature. Clin Exp Rheum 2001;19(Suppl 24):S55-S58
(170) Rizvi SW, McGrath Jr H. The therapeutic effect of cigarette smoking on oral/ genital aphthosis and other manifestations of Behçet's disease (letter). Clin Exp Rheum 2001;19(Suppl 24):S77-S78
(171) Orem A, Deger O, Cimsit G, Karahan SC, Akyol N, Yildirmis S. Plasma lipoprotein(a) and its relationship with disease activity in patients with Behçet's disease. Eur J Clin Chem Clin Biochem 1995; 33(No 8):473-78
(172) Orem A, Cimsit G, Deger O, Vanizor A, Karahan SC. Autoantibodies against oxidatively modified low-density lipoprotein in patients with Behçet's disease. Dermatology 1999:198:243-46
(173) Erem C, Uslu T, Deger O, Tosun M, Kavgaci H. Increased plasma lipoprotein(a) concentrations in Behçet's disease and its relation to vascular events. Heart 2000;84:208 (Scientific Letters)
(174) Plotkin GR. Pulmonary Involvement (Miscellaneous Clinical Manifestations, Part 1) in Behçet's Disease: A Contemporary Synopsis. Plotkin G, Calabro J and O'Duffy JD (eds), c1988 Futura Publishing, NY; p220
(175) Lee, Bang, Lee and Sohn (eds), Behçet's Disease: A Guide to its Clinical Understanding. Copyright 2001 Springer-Verlag, Germany, p20
(176) Papiris SA, Moutsopoulos HM. Rare rheumatic disorders. A. Behçet's disease. Baillieres Clin Rheumatol 1993 Feb;7(1):173-8
(177) Raz I, Okon E, Chajek-Shaul T. Pulmonary manifestations in Behçet's syndrome. Chest 1989 Mar;95(3):585-9
(178) Dilsen N, Cavdar T, Aral O, Konice M, Erkan F and Ocal L. Pulmonary Involvement in Behçet's Disease in Turkey. In Behçet's Disease: Basic and Clinical Aspects. O'Duffy JD, Kokmen E (eds.), Marcel Dekker, c1991, p220-225
(179) Mead S, Kidd D, Good C, Plant G. Behçet's syndrome may present with partial seizures. J Neurol Neurosurg Psychiatry 2000;68:392-393 (March)
(180) Lueck CJ, Pires M, McCartney AC, Graham EM. Ocular and neurological Behçet's disease without orogenital ulceration? J Neurology Neurosurg Psych. 1993, 56:505-8
(181) Matsuo T, Itami M, Nakagawa H, Nagayama M. The incidence and pathology of conjunctival ulceration in Behçet's syndrome. Brit J of Ophth

2002;86:140-3

(182) Cooper C, Pippard EC, Wickham C, Chamberlain MA, Barker DJ. Is Behçet's disease triggered by childhood infection? Ann Rheum Dis 1989;48:421-423

(183) Isogai E, Yokota K, Fujii N et al."Characterization and functional properties of streptococcus sanguis isolated from patients with Behçet's disease. In "Behçet's Disease," c1993 Elsevier Science Publishers BV, Godeau and Wechsler (eds), p73-82

(184) Lee ES, Lee S, Bang D, Cho YH, Sohn S. Detection of herpes simplex virus DNA by polymerase chain reaction in saliva of patients with Behçet's disease. In "Behçet's Disease", c1993 Elsevier Science Publishers BV, Godeau and Wechsler (Eds.), pp83-86

(185) Lehner T. Advances in the immunopathogenesis of Behçet's disease. In "Behçet's Disease: A Guide to its Clinical Understanding", c2001 Springer-Verlag Berlin Heidelberg. Lee, Bang, Lee and Sohn (Eds.), pp3-4

(186) Ergun T, Ince U et al. HSP 60 expression in mucocutaneous lesions of Behçet's disease. J Am Acad Dermatol 2001 Dec;45(6):904-9

(187) Evereklioglu C, Cokkeser Y, Doganay S, Er H, Kizilay A. Audio-vestibular evaluation in patients with Behçet's syndrome. J Laryngol Otol 2001 Sep;115(9):704-8

(188) Lee, Bang, Lee and Sohn (Eds). Behçet's Disease: A Guide to its Clinical Understanding. Springer Verlag, Berlin, c2001, p 76

(189) Chang HK, Kim JU. The study of HLA antigens in familial Behçet's disease. Yonsei Med J, 2000;41:3 (Suppl), p36

(190) Calamia K, Mazlumzadeh M, Balabanova M, Bagheri M, O'Duffy JD. Clinical characteristics of United States patients with Behçet's disease. Yonsei Med J, 2000;41:3 (Suppl), p 9

(191) Akpolat T, Koc Y, Yeniay I, Akpek G et al. Familial Behçet's disease. Eur J Med 1992 Nov;1(7):391-5

(192) Koptagel_ital G, Tuncer O, Enbiyaoglu G, Bayramoglu Z. A psychosomatic investigation of Behçet's disease. Psychother Psychosom 1983;40(1-4):263-71

(193) Cengiz K, Ozkan A. Psychiatric aspects of complete Behçet's syndrome: review of fifteen cases. In "Behçet's Disease: Basic and Clinical Aspects." O'Duffy JD, Kokmen E (Eds.), c1991 Marcel Dekker, NY, p115-118

(194) Achiron A, Noy S, Krause I, Yosipovitch G, Wysenbeek A, Weinberger A. Neuropsychiatric evaluation of asymptomatic patients with Behçet's disease. In "Behçet's Disease." Godeau P, Wechslet B (Eds.) c1993 Elsevier Science Publishers BV, p435-38

(195) Calikoglu E, Onder M, Cosar B, Candansayar S. Depression, anxiety levels and general psychological profile in Behçet's disease. Dermatology 2001;203(3):238-40

(196) Dilsen G, Sendil G, Onk A, Onen L, Yaliman A et al. A psychological assessment of Behçet's disease. In "Behçet's Disease." Godeau P, Wechslet B (Eds.) c1993 Elsevier Science Publishers BV, p439-42

(197) Yamada M, Kashiwamura K, Nakamura Y, Ota T, Nakamura K. On psychiatric symptoms of neuro-Behçet's syndrome. Folia Psychiatr Neurol Jpn 1978;32(2):191-7

(198) Oktem-Tanor O, Baykan-Kurt B, Gurvit IH, Akman-Demir G, Serdaroglu P. Neuropsychological follow-up of 12 patients with neuro-Behcet disease. J Neurol 1999 Feb;246(2):113-9

(199) Faraf S, Al-Shubaili A, Montaser A, Hussein JM et al. Behçet's syndrome: a report of 41 patients with emphasis on neurological manifestations. J Neurol Neurosurg Psychiatry 1998;64:382-384

(200) Zafirakis P, Foster CS. Adamantiades-Behcet Disease in "Diagnosis and Treatment of Uveitis." c2002 WB Saunders Co, Foster and Vitale (Eds.), p632-652

(201) Apaydin S, Erek E, Ulku U, Hamuryudan V, Yazici H, Sariyar M. A success-ful renal transplantation in Behçet's syndrome. Ann Rheum Dis 1999 Novem-ber;58:719

(202) Akpolat T, Akkoyunlu M, Akpolat I, Dilek M, Odabas AR, Ozen S. Renal Behçet's disease: A cumulative analysis. Semin Arthritis Rheum 2002

Apr;31(5):317-37

(203) Zivkovic S, Markovic D, Petrovic S. [Caries incidence in rheumatic patients.] [Article in Serbo-Croatian]. Stomatol Glas Srb 1989 Jun-Aug;36(3):239-47

(204) Sacks, O. "Migraine Aura and Hallucinatory Constants" in "Migraine." c1992 Vintage Books, NY, p276, 280

(205) Lehner T, Barnes CG. "Diagnosis and Classification of Behçet's Syndrome" in "Behçet's Syndrome: Clinical and Immunological Features." c1979 Academic Press, London; Lehner and Barnes (Eds.), p6

(206) Diri E, Mat C, Hamuryudan V, Yurdakul S et al. Papulopustular skin lesions are seen more frequently in patients with Behçet's syndrome who have arthritis: a controlled and masked study. Ann Rheum Dis 2001 November;60:1074-76

(207) Roux H, Richard P, Arrighi A, Bergaoui N. [Autochthonous behcet's disease. Apropos of 73 cases][{Article in French]. Rev Rhum Mal Osteoartic 1989 Apr;56(5):383-8

(208) Davatchi F, Shahram F, Akbarian M et al. Classification tree for the diagnosis of Behçet's disease. In "Behçet's Disease" c1993 Elsevier Science Publishers, Wechsler and Godeau (Eds.), p245-248

(209) Shimokawabe K, Ishikawa S, Fukuda T, Fukushima K. Central autonomic dysfunction in patients with Behçet's disease examined by sleep polygraphy. In "Behçet's Disease: Basic and Clinical Aspects", c1991 Marcel Dekker, O'Duffy and Kokmen (Eds.), p125-126

(210) Gulekon A, Atik L, Isik E, Gurer MA, Arikan Z. Sleep pattern in Behçet's disease. In "Behçet's Disease" c1993 Elsevier Science Publishers, Wechsler and Godeau (Eds.), p447-449

(211) Schiff S, Moffatt R, Mandel W, Rubin S. Acute myocardial infarction and recurrent ventricular arrhythmias in Behçet's syndrome. American Heart Journal, March 1982, p438-440

(212) Assaad-Khalil S, Sobhy M, Abou-Seif M, El-Sawy M. Cardiac manifestations of Behçet's disease: clinical, genetic and echocardiographic study. In "Behçet's Disease" c1993 Elsevier Science Publishers, Wechsler and Godeau (Eds.), p481-86

(213) Morelli S, Perrone C, Ferrante L, Sgreccia A et al. Cardiac involvement in Behçet's disease. Cardiology 1997;88:513-517

(214) Mirone L, Altomonte L, Ferlisi EM, Zoli A, Magaro M. Behçet's disease and cardiac arrhythmias. Clinical rheumatology 1997;16, No. 1, p99-100

(215) Goldeli O, Ural D, Komsuoglu B et al. Abnormal QT dispersion in Behçet's disease. Int J Cardiol 1997 Aug 29;61(1):55-9

(216) Dilsen G, Oral A, Aydin R, Sabuncu H. Autonomic dysfunction in Behçet's disease. In "Behçet's Disease: Basic and Clinical Aspects", c1991 Marcel Dekker, O'Duffy and Kokmen (Eds.), p127-132

(217) Aksoyek S, Aytemir K, Ozer N, Ozcebe O, Oto A. Assessment of autonomic nervous system function in patients with Behçet's disease by spectral analysis of heart rate variability. J Auton Nerv Syst 1999 Sep 24;77(2-3):190-4

(218) Rogers III RS. "Recurrent aphthous stomatitis in the diagnosis of Behçet's disease." In "Behçet's Disease: A Guide to its Clinical Understanding." Lee, Bang, Lee and Sohn (Eds). Springer Verlag, Berlin, c2001, pp119-128

(219) Kahn MA. Review and management consideration of recurrent aphthous stomatitis and Behçet's disease. ABDA Patient/Family Conference presentation, October 2001, Boston, MA.

(220) Foster CS. Personal communication, and "Adamantiades-Behcet Disease" in "Diagnosis and Treatment of Uveitis." Foster and Vitale (Eds.), c.2002, WB Saunders, p632

(221) Jensen L. Personal communication, May 2002

(222) Plotkin GR. "Genitourinary involvement" in "Behçet's Disease: A Contemporary Synopsis," Plotkin, Calabro and O'Duffy (Eds), c1988 Futura Publishing, p256

(223) Assaad-Khalil SH. "Clinical, genetic, immunological, and biochemical features of 180 Egyptian patients with Behçet's disease." In "Behçet's Disease: Basic and Clinical Aspects," O'Duffy JD and Kokmen E (Eds.), c1991 Marcel Dekker, p273

(224) Calamia KT, Mazlumzadeh M, Balabanova M, Bagheri M, O'Duffy JD. Clinical characteristics of United States patients with Behçet's disease. Yonsei Medical Journal June 2000;Vol 41 Supp., p9

(225) Gul A et al. Lack of association of HLA-B51 with a severe disease course in Behçet's disease. Rheumatology (Oxford) 2001 June;40(6):668-72

(226) Namba K, Ogawa T, Inaba G, Kishi I, Miyanaga Y. Two cases of Behçet's disease with Sjogren's syndrome. In "Behçet's Disease," Wechsler and Godeau (Eds.), c1993 Elsevier Science Publishers BV, pp299-302

(227) Lee S, Bang D, Lee ES, Sohn S. Table 3: Clinical manifestations of Adamantiades-Behçet's disease in different countries. In" Behçet's Disease: A Guide to its Clinical Understanding," c2001 Springer-Verlag, p20

(228) Benamour S, Zeroual B, Alaoui FZ. Joint manifestations in Behçet's disease. A review of 340 cases. Rev Rhum Engl Ed 1998 May;65(5):299-307

(229) Lee S, Bang D. Joint manifestations. In "Behcet Disease," eMedicine Journal, July 10 2001;2(7):p7

(230) Schirmer M, Calamia KT, Direskeneli H. Ninth international conference on Behçet's disease, Seoul, Korea, May 27-29, 2000. J of Rheumatology 2001;28(3):636-39

(231) El-Ramahi KM, Al-Dalaan A, Al-Balaa S, Al-Kawi MZ, Bohlega S. Joint fluid analysis in Behcet disease. In "Behçet's Disease," Wechsler and Godeau (Eds.), c1993 Elsevier Science Publishers BV, pp279-282

(232) O'Duffy JD, Carney A, Deodhar S. Behçet's disease: report of 10 cases, three with new manifestations. Ann Intern Med 1971;75:561-70

(233) Hagiwara N, Harashima S, Tukamoto H, Horiuchi T. [A case of Behçet's disease with chronic and repeated sudden hearing loss: successful treatment with intravenous cyclophosphamide pulse therapy.][Japanese] Ryumachi 2001 Oct;41(5):858-63

(234) Tellioglu T, Robertson D. Orthostatic intolerance in Behçet's disease. Autonomic Neuroscience: Basic and clinical 89 (2001):96-99

(235) Plotkin GR. "Gastrointestinal features" in "Behçet's Disease: A Contemporary Synopsis," Plotkin, Calabro and O'Duffy (Eds), c1988 Futura Publishing, p240

(236) Yashiro K, Nagasako K, et al. Esophageal lesions in intestinal Behçet's disease. Endoscopy 1986 Mar;18(2):57-60

(237) Kasahara Y, Tanaka S, et al. Intestinal involvement in Behçet's disease: review of 136 surgical cases in the Japanese literature. Dis Colon Rectum 1981;24:103-106

(238) Plotkin GR. "Gastrointestinal features" in "Behçet's Disease: A Contemporary Synopsis," Plotkin, Calabro and O'Duffy (Eds), c1988 Futura Publishing, p248

(239) Chung SY, Ha HK, Kim JH et al. Radiologic findings of Behcet syndrome involving the gastrointestinal tract. Radiographics 2001 Jul-Aug;21(4):911-24

(240) Bayraktar Y, Ozaslan E, Van Thiel DH. Gastrointestinal manifestations of Behçet's disease. J Clin Gastroenterol 2000 Mar;30(2):144-54

(241) Zeis J. "Patti and Brandon" in "You Are Not Alone: 15 People with Behçet's." c1997, p42

(242) Gubbins PO, Bertch KE. Drug absorption in gastrointestinal disease and surgery. Clinical pharmacokinetic and therapeutic implications. Clin Pharmacokinet 1991 Dec;21(6):431-47

(243) McCallum RW, George SJ. Gastric dysmotility and gastroparesis. 1092-8472 2001 Apr;4(2):179-191

(244) Forster J, Sarosiek I et al. Gastric pacing is a new surgical treatment for gastroparesis. Am J Surg 2001 Dec;182(6):676-81

(245) Kennedy NB. "The Melungeons: The Resurrection of a Proud People." Mercer Univ Press, GA, c.1997. Introduction.

CHAPTER 2

Treatment for Behçet's Disease

Disclaimer: The author of this book is not medically trained. Any information provided here is meant to support, and not replace, the relationship that exists between a patient and his/her health care provider. Please speak with your doctor before making any changes to your treatment plan. Parents are warned that medications and dosages (where listed) are set at adult levels, and should not be considered safe or appropriate for a child's treatment without first speaking to a physician. Pregnant or lactating patients must check each drug's safety with their physician prior to use. The contents of this chapter have been carefully screened, but cannot be guaranteed for completeness or accuracy.

Treatment for Behçet's Disease Sorted by Medication

The following table is copyright 1999 Massachusetts Medical Society. All rights reserved. Reprinted with permission. Sakane T, Takeno M, Suzuki N, Inaba G. Behçet's disease. *New Engl J Med 1999;341:1289 (Table 3)*

TREATMENT	Dose	Used as First-Line Therapy	Used as Alternative Therapy
Triamcinolone acetonide ointment [Kenalog]	3 times/ day topically	Oral ulcers	
Betamethasone ointment	3 times/ day topically	Genital ulcers	
Betamethasone drops	1-2 drops 3 times daily topically	Anterior uveitis, retinal vasculitis	
Dexamethasone [Decadron]	1.0-1.5 mg injected below Tenon's capsule for ocular attack	Retinal vasculitis	
Prednisolone	5-20 mg/day orally		Erythema nodosum, anterior uveitis, retinal vasculitis

57

Treatment	Dose	Used as First-Line Therapy	Used as Alternative Therapy
Prednisolone	20-100 mg /day orally	Gastrointestinal lesions, acute meningoencephalitis, chronic progressive central nervous system lesions, arteritis	Retinal vasculitis, venous thrombosis
Methylprednisolone	1000 mg/day for 3 days IV	Acute meningoencephalitis, chronic progressive central nervous system lesions, arteritis	Gastrointestinal lesions, venous thrombosis
Tropicamide drops	1-2 drops once or twice a day topically	Anterior uveitis	
Tetracycline	250 mg in water solution once a day topically	Oral ulcers	
Colchicine	0.5-1.5 mg/day orally [JZ: standard dose is 0.6-1.2 mg/day]	Oral ulcers,* genital ulcers,* pseudo-folliculitis,* erythema nodosum, anterior uveitis, retinal vasculitis	Arthritis
Thalidomide	100-300 mg /day orally	Oral ulcers,* genital ulcers, * pseudofolliculitis *	
Dapsone	100 mg /day		Oral ulcers, genital ulcers, pseudofolliculitis, erythema nodosum
Pentoxifylline [JZ: brand-name **Trental** works best over generic]	300 mg/day orally [JZ- standard dose is 3 x 400 mg/day orally]		Oral ulcers, genital ulcers, pseudofolliculitis, erythema nodosum
Azathioprine [Imuran]	100 mg/day orally		Retinal vasculitis,* arthritis,* chronic progressive central nervous system lesions, arteritis, venous thrombosis
Chlorambucil [Leukeran]	5 mg/day orally		Retinal vasculitis, * acute meningoencephalitis, chronic progressive CNS lesions, arteritis, venous thrombosis

Treatment	Dose	Used as First-Line Therapy	Used as Alternative Therapy
Cyclophos-phamide [Cytoxan]	50-100 mg /day orally		Retinal vasculitis, acute meningoence-phalitis, chronic progressive CNS lesions, arteritis, venous thrombosis
	700-1000 mg /mo IV		Retinal vasculitis, acute meningoence-phalitis, chronic progressive CNS lesions, arteritis, venous thrombosis
Methotrexate	7.5-15 mg/wk orally		Retinal vasculitis, arthritis, chronic progressive CNS lesions
Cyclosporine ++	5 mg/kg of body weight/day orally	Retinal vasculitis *	
Interferon alfa	5 millionU/day IM or SC		Retinal vasculitis, arthritis
Indomethacin [Indocin]	50-75 mg/day orally	Arthritis	
Sulfasalazine [Azulfidine]	1-3 g/day orally	Gastrointestinal lesions	Arthritis
Warfarin +++	2-10 mg/day orally	Venous thrombosis	Arteritis
Heparin +++	5000-20,000 U/day SC	Venous thrombosis	Arteritis
Aspirin #	50-100 mg/day orally	Arteritis, venous thrombosis	Chronic progressive CNS lesions
Dipyridamole [Persantine]	300 mg/day orally	Arteritis, venous thrombosis	Chronic progressive CNS lesions
Surgery	——		Gastrointestinal lesions, arteritis, venous thrombosis

Data are from Kastner,[1] Kaklamani et al,[2] Nussenblatt,[3] Miyachi et al,[31] Hamuryudan et al.,[32,33] Yasui et al.,[34] O'Duffy et al.,[35,36] Kazokoglu et al.,[37] Masuda et al.,[38] Kotake et al.,[39] Zouboulis and Orfanos,[40] and Lee et al.[41] **IV** denotes intravenously, **IM** intramuscularly, and **SC** subcutaneously.

* The efficacy of this drug for this use has been reported in controlled clinical trials.

++   Cyclosporine is contraindicated in patients with acute meningoence-phalitis or chronic progressive central nervous system lesions.

+++   This drug should be used with caution in patients with pulmonary vascular lesions.

\#   Low-dose aspirin is used as an antiplatelet agent.

References for above table:
1) Kastner DL. Intermittent and periodic arthritic syndromes. In: Koopman WJ, ed. Arthritis and allied conditions: a textbook of rheumatology. 13th ed. Vol. 1. Baltimore: Williams & Wilkins, 1997:1279-306
2) Kaklamani VG, Variopoulos G, Kaklamanis PG. Behçet's disease. Semin Arthritis Rheum 1998;27:197-217
3) Nussenblatt RB. Uveitis in Behçet's disease. Int Rev Immunol 1997;14:67-79
31) Miyachi Y, Taniguchi S, Ozaki M, Horio T. Colchicine in the treatment of the cutaneous manifestations of Behçet's disease. Br J Dermatol 1981;104:67-9
32) Hamuryudan V, Mat C, Saip S, et al. Thalidomide in the treatment of the mucocutaneous lesions of the Behcet syndrome: a randomized, double-blind, placebo-controlled trial. Ann Intern Med 1998;128:443-50
33) Hamuryudan V, Ozyazgan Y, Hizli N, et al. Azathioprine in Behçet's syndrome: effects on long-term prognosis. Arthritis Rheum 1997;40:769-74
34) Yasui K, Ohta K, Kobayashi M, Aizawa T, Komiyama A. Successful treatment of Behcet disease with pentoxifylline. Ann Intern Med 1996;124:891-3
35) O'Duffy JD, Robertson DM, Goldstein NP. Chlorambucil in the treatment of uveitis and menigoencephalitis of Behçet's disease. Am J Med 1984;76:75-84
36) O'Duffy JD, Calamia K, Cohen S, et al. Interferon-alpha treatment of Behçet's disease. J Rheumatol 1998;25:1938-44
37) Kazokoglu H, Saatci O, Cuhadaroglu H, Eldem B. Long-term effects of cyclophosphamide and colchicine treatment in Behçet's disease. Ann Ophthalmol 1991;23:148-51
38) Masuda K, Nakajima A, Urayama A, Nakae K, Kogure M, Inaba G. Double-masked trial of cyclosporin versus colchicine and long-term open study of cyclosporin in Behçet's disease. Lancet 1989;1:1093-6
39) Kotake S, Higashi K, Yoshikawa K, Sasamoto Y, Okamoto T, Matsuda H. Central nervous system symptoms in patients with Behcet disease receiving cyclosporine therapy. Ophthalmology 1999;106:586-9
40) Zouboulis CC, Orafanos CE. Treatment of Adamantiades-Behcet disease with systemic interferon alfa. Arch Dermatol 1998;134:1010-6
41) Lee KS, Kim SJ, Lee BC, Yoon DS, Lee WJ, Chi HS. Surgical treatment of intestinal Behçet's disease. Yonsei Med J 1997;38:455-60

Treatment for Behçet's Disease
Sorted by Symptoms or Related Health Issues

Disclaimer: The author of this book is not medically trained. Any information provided here is meant to support, and not replace, the relationship that exists between a patient and his/her health care provider. Listed medications may not be safe or appropriate for children. Pregnant or lactating patients must discuss each drug's safety with their physician(s) prior to use. **This section is only a sampling of the total medications available to treat each symptom, and the drugs shown may not be appropriate for your specific medical condition.** Please speak with your physician or health care provider in advance about all possible treatments, and the dosages, side effects, and drug interactions associated with each one. Do not change your treatment plan based solely on the information in this chapter. The use of medication trade names should not be considered an endorsement. **Even though a symptom or health issue is listed here, it does not mean that you will personally experience that particular problem. Some listed health problems are not directly related to Behçet's disease, but are included because of anecdotal accounts from BD patients who have experienced the symptoms.** Medications are listed first by trade name, and then by generic name in parentheses. Medications and products were suggested through medical journal articles, and through personal recommendations from physicians, health care providers and other patients. References for this section can be found at the end of the chapter.

Aphthous ulcerations (oral)
(Additional oral treatments can be found at the end of this chapter)
Local anesthetics: Ambesol; Lidocaine Viscous 2%; TOPEX; Zetacaine metered spray; Lidex gel 0.05%
Other treatments: Carmex ointment; Orabase; Dr. Tichenor's mouthwash diluted 3:1; Magic Mouthwash or Bilson's Solution (ingredients on page 22); Zilactin; Aphthasol (amlexanox) 5% paste; Kenalog in Orabase; Peridex mouth rinse; Difflam mouth rinse; tetracycline rinse; colchicine; Trental (brand name only); dapsone; Ergamisol; prednisone; thalidomide

Aphthous ulcerations (genital)
Local anesthetics: Vagisil; Baby Orajel with a covering of Vaseline prior to urinating; Lidocaine Viscous 2%, Instillagel (clinimed); ELA-Max 5 (5% lidocaine); EMLA cream; Liquidcaine; Sustaine Blue Gel
Other treatments: Preparation H; urination through an empty toilet tissue tube after application of Vaseline to prevent splashing of urine on ulcers; Lidex (fluocinomide); Bactroban (mupirocin); Sigmacort (hydrocortisone acetate); Kenacomb cream/ointment; Mycolog cream/ointment; Elocon cream; Peridex applied genitally; Kenalog paste; colchicine; Trental (brand name only); dapsone; Ergamisol; prednisone; cyclosporine; interferon alpha-2A; Imuran; CellCept (mycophenolate mofetil); Remicade (infliximab); Enbrel (etanercept); thalidomide

Dry mouth
Salagen (pilocarpine hydrochloride)
Evoxac (cevimeline)
Dry Mouth Relief by Natrol (anhydrous crystalline maltose)

Esophageal spasms
(muscle relaxants)
Baclofen (lioresal)
Flexeril (cyclobenzaprine)
Valium (diazepam)

Fatigue, BD-associated
(with or without depression)
Dexedrine (dextroamphetamine sulfate)
Prozac (fluoxetine)

Fatigue (continued):
Ritalin (methylphenidate hydrochloride)
Trental (pentoxifylline): anecdotal reports strongly suggest use of
    non-generic (i.e. Trental)
Tricyclic anti-depressants (e.g. Elavil) combined with SSRIs (e.g. Prozac or
    Zoloft)
Wellbutrin (bupropion)
Zoloft (sertraline)

Folliculitis
Topical corticosteroids
Avlosulfon (dapsone)
colchicine
thalidomide
Trental (pentoxifylline): anecdotal reports strongly suggest use of
    non-generic (i.e. Trental)

Gastroesophageal reflux (GERD)
Carafate (sucralfate)
Prevacid (lansoprazole)
Prilosec (omeprazole)
Tagamet (cimetidine)

Gastrointestinal involvement
Asacol (mesalamine) : treats and maintains remission of ulcerative colitis
Bentyl (dicyclomine hydrochloride) : treats ulcers, hypermotility & GI tract
    spasms associated w/ colitis
Carafate (sucralfate) : anti-ulcer drug; Carafate suspension used for oral/
    esophageal ulcers
Lomotil (diphenoxylate hydrochloride with atropine sulfate) : treats diarrhea
Medrol (methylprednisolone)
prednisone
Prevacid (lansoprazole) : heals ulcers; healing & relief of erosive esophagitis
Remicade (infliximab) : classed as a treatment for Crohn's disease
Sulfasalazine (azulfidine) : used in treatment of colitis, Crohn's disease
Future possibilities (undergoing clinical trials) :
    CDP571 ; Antegren (natalizumab)

Headaches, vascular
Catapres (clonidine) : also used for ulcerative colitis, neuralgia
Corgard (nadolol)
Depakote (divalproex sodium)
Inderal (propranolol) : also treats cardiac arrhythmias, performance anxiety
Periactin (cyproheptadine) : also used for generalized itching, allergic
    conjunctivitis, Cushing's syndrome
Sansert (methysergide maleate)

Hearing loss
cortisone (high dose)
cyclosporine A
Cytoxan (cyclophosphamide) high dose IV Methylprednisolone (pulse-dose)
Topamax

Itching: overall body
(oral medications)
Atarax 25 mg (hydroxyzine hydrochloride)
Zyrtec (cetirizine hydrochloride)

Meningoencephalitis, acute
prednisolone
Medrol (methylprednisolone)
Chlorambucil (leukeran)
Cytoxan (cyclophosphamide)

Nausea
Compazine (prochlorperazine)
Phenergan (promethazine hydrochloride)
Zofran (ondansetron hydrochloride): caution - very expensive

Neuro-Behçet's, progressive
CellCept (mycophenolate mofetil)
Chlorambucil (leukeran)
Cytoxan (cyclophosphamide)
Imuran (azathioprine)
Medrol (methylprednisolone)
methotrexate (low dose, weekly) followed with folic acid to reduce nausea
Persantine (dipyridamole)
prednisone

Pain: joint pain/ arthritis
Over-the-counter NSAIDS and analgesics (e.g. Advil, Aleve; Excedrin, Tylenol)
Arava (leflunomide)
Celebrex (celecoxib)
colchicine
corticosteroids (e.g. Prednisone, Decadron, Medrol, Aristocort)
Enbrel (etanercept)
Feldene (piroxicam)
Interferon alpha-2a
Neoral or Sandimmune (cyclosporine)
Plaquenil (hydroxychloroquine)
Remicade (infliximab): caution - expensive; may not be covered by insurance
Rheumatrex (methotrexate)
Sulfasalazine (azulfidine)
Vioxx (rofecoxib) *[JZ-an article in **Arch Intern Med** 2002;162(6):713-715
described five cases of aseptic meningitis linked to the use of this
medication]*

Pain: migraine-specific meds
Excedrin Migraine / Extra-strength Excedrin
Imitrex (sumatriptan succinate)
Relpax (eletriptan)
Topamax (topiramate)
Valproate (depakote)
Zomig (zolmitriptan)

Pain: severe/ chronic
Duragesic (fentanyl skin patch)
Fioricet or Tylenol 2,3,4 (acetaminophen with codeine)
Lortab or Vicodin (hydrocodone with acetaminophen)
Medtronic internal morphine pump, delivers via spinal cord
Methadone (dolophine)
MS Contin (morphine sulfate)
Neurontin or Pregabalin (gabapentin)
OxyContin (oxycodone)
Percocet (acetaminoophen with oxycodone)
Sublimaze (fentanyl)
Toradol (ketorolac tromethamine)
Ultram (tramadol)

Raynaud's phenomenon
Capoten (captopril)

Restless legs syndrome
Klonopin (clonazepam)
Mirapex (pramipexole)
Neurontin (gabapentin)
Tegretol (carbamazepine)

Skin lesions / rashes
Over-the-counter corticosteroid creams
Avlosulfon (dapsone) : oral tablets
Bactroban ointment (mupirocin 2%)
CellCept (mycophenolate mofetil) : oral tablets
Cleocin 1% (clindamycin)
Elocon (mometasone furoate)
Interferon alpha-2a
Mycolog II (nystatin and Triamcinolone acetonide)
Silvadene cream 1% (silver sulfadiazine)
Temovate (clobetasol)
Trental (pentoxifylline) : oral tablets. Use **non-generic** (i.e. Trental)

Sleep aids - for occasional use
Ambien (zolpidem tartrate)
Benadryl (diphenhydramine)
Flexeril (cyclobenzaprine)
Sonata (zaleplon) - can be taken during the night without next-morning effects
Trazodone

Sore/ swollen throat
flurbiprofen 8.75mg lozenges *[JZ: See Benrimoj SI et al. Efficacy and
        tolerability of the anti-inflammatory throat lozenge flurbiprofen
        8.75mg in the treatment of sore throat. Clin Drug Invest 21(3):183-93*

Uveitis/ retinal vasculitis
CellCept (mycophenolate mofetil)
Corticosteroids — topical drops/ oral/ injected *[JZ: Toker et al, in the Brit J
        Ophth 2002 May;86(5):521-3 indicate that high-dose intravenous
        steroid therapy is effective in controlling severe, acute posterior*

Uveitis / retinal vasculitis (continued)
uveitis in BD patients.]

Cytoxan (cyclophosphamide)

Combination therapy of low-dose pulse cyclophosphamide and methotrexate Combination therapy of cyclosporin-A, prednisone and methotrexate

Interferon alpha-2a [JZ: has also been found useful in treatment of retinal neovascularisation: See Stuebiger N et al, Complete regression of retinal neovascularisation after therapy with interferon alfa in Behçet's disease.Br J Ophth 2000;84:1432 (December)]

Imuran (azathioprine)

Leukeran (chlorambucil)

Neoral or Sandimmune (cyclosporine) : pentoxifylline can be used simultaneously to combat potential renal problems associated with cyclosporine

Prograf (tacrolimus - FK506) : do not use in combination with cyclosporine

Remicade (infliximab): expensive; health insurance may not cover cost

Zenapax (daclizumab) : undergoing clinical trials at National Eye Institute for treatment of BD-related eye inflammation

Future treatment options
The following medications/treatments are in various clinical trial stages:

1) Envision (R) (created by Control Delivery Systems of Watertown, MA, in conjunction with Bausch & Lomb) is a small capsule that is implanted within the eye to control problems such as uveitis and age-related macular degeneration. The implant contains steroids or cyclosporine in controlled-release dosages that can last for years. It has the advantage of delivering necessary medicine to the specific area that needs it, without the systemic side effects that can result from taking these drugs orally or through injections. In clinical trials, some patients have experienced increased eye pressure (glaucoma) from the implants, or infection from the surgical incision; however the developer states that if these problems occur, they can be corrected with other currently available medications. Control Delivery Systems expects to extend the usefulness of this technology into other areas, such as the relief of joint pain through similar implants.

2) Veldona (R) (produced by Amarillo Biosciences in Amarillo, TX, in conjunction with Atrix Laboratories, CO) is **low-dose oral interferon-alpha lozenges.** Anecdotal reports of results in "compassionate-use" patients are very encouraging, with a marked reduction in symptoms, and a virtual absence of side effects compared to injectable versions of interferon; may not be as effective if preceded by methotrexate tx. More info on Veldona can be found at www.amarbio.com. The FDA gave Veldona orphan drug status in October 2001 for the treatment of Behçet's disease.

3) IV Lidocaine: on 5/10/02, Reuters Medical News reported that fibromyalgia (FM) patients non-responsive to standard treatments may benefit from an intravenous infusion of the anesthetic lignocaine (Lidocaine). JH Raphael, MD of the Dudley Group of Hospitals in West Midlands UK, found that FM patients in his pilot study experienced significant reductions in depression, dependency on others, median pain scores, and ability to cope. Randomized controlled trials are planned.

Various Management Therapies for
Oral Ulcerations and Related Complications

This listing is reprinted with permission of Michael A. Kahn, DDS, from presentation handouts at the American Behçet's Disease Association Patient and Family Conference, October 2001, Boston, MA. Dr. Kahn's listing is a compilation of information from many sources, including medical research journals, anecdotal reports, and internet resources. Do not change your treatment plan, or begin taking any of these medications for the treatment of oral ulcerations or related complications without first meeting with your primary care physician.

Antianxiety/Antidepressant
Diazepam (Valium)
Phenelzine (Nardil): antidepressant (monoamine oxidase inhibitor)

Antibiotics/Antimicrobials/Antibacterial oral rinse
Cefaclor (Ceclor)
Chlorhexidine digluconate (Peridex)
Dapsone (Avlosulfon)
Metronidazole (Flagyl)
Minocycline hydrochloride (Minocin)
Topical and liquid tetracyclines (Achromycin)

Antifungals
Clotrimazole (Mycelex)
Gentian violet
Griseofulvin (Grisactin)
Ketoconazole (Nizoral)
Miconazole (Micatin)
Nystatin (Mycostatin

Antihistamine/Antacid
Azelastine (Astelin)
Diphenhydramine Hydrochloride (Benadryl)
Magnesium Hydroxide (Philips Milk of Magnesia)

Antineoplastic
Chlorambucil (Leukeran)
Cyclophosphamide (Cytoxan)
 Methotrexate (Rheumatrex)
Interferon alpha-2a (Roferon-A) and alpha-2c
Tretinoin (Retin-A)-retinoic acid derivative

Diet Supplements
Cultured buttermilk
Folic acid
Iron
L-lysine
Vitamin A
Vitamin B12
Yogurt (active cultures of Lactobacillus acidophilus and Lactobacillus bulgaricus)
Zinc sulfate

Immune Enhancers
Immune Globulin (Gammastan)
Levamisole hydrochloride (Ergamisol)
LongoVital

Transfer factor
Viral vaccines

Immunosuppressants/Anti-Inflammatory/Corticosteroid
Amlexanox paste 5% (Aphthasol)
Azathioprine (Imuran)
Betamethasone (Diprolene)
Betamethasone valerate (Valisone)
Clobetasol proprionate (Temovate(r)) Colchicine (Colchiquim(r)) Cyclosporine (Sandimmune)
Dexamethasone elixir (Decadron)
Fluocinonide (Lidex)
Flumethasone pivalate (Locorten)
Hydrocortisone sodium succinate (Orabase HCA)
Methylprednisolone (Medrol)
Prednisolone (Prelone)
Prednisone (Deltasone)
Tacrolimus (Prograf)
Triamcinolone acetonide (Kenalog)

Local Anesthetics
Benzydamine hydrochloride
Dyclonine hydrochloride (Dyclone)
Lidocaine (Xylocaine)
Tetracaine (Pontocaine)

Protective pastes, aseptics, astringents, cauterizers, and mouthwashes
Carbamide peroxide (Gly-oxide)
Carbenoxolone sodium mouthwash
Carboxymethylcellulose
Cyanoacrylate
Hydrogen peroxide
Hydroxypropylcellulose
Listerine mouthwash
Silver nitrate (Negatan)
Tannic acid (Zilactin)
Thermal cauterization
OTC medicaments-benzocaine, camphor, phenol, menthol, eugenol

Others
Attapulgite (Kaopectate) - antidiarrheal
Chlorgan
Cryosurgery
Disodium cromoglycate
Enhanced salivary peroxidase
Estrogen replacement
Hydroxychloroquine sulfate (Plaquenil) - antimalarial
Hypnosis
Laser
Pentoxifylline (Trental) - blood viscosity reducer agent
Alprostadil Prostaglandin E1 - prostaglandin
Sucralfate (Carafate) - gastrointestinal agent
Thalidomide
X-ray therapy

Sources used in the compilation of
Treatment for Behcet's Disease, Sorted by Symptom:
--Yonsei Medical Journal June 2000:41(3) Supplement. Ninth International

Conference on Behçet's Disease, May 2000, Korea; p1-53
--Restless Legs Syndrome Foundation, Medical Bulletin September 2001 at www.rls.org
--Russell AI, Lawson WA and Haskard DO. Potential new therapeutic options in Behçet's syndrome. BioDrugs 2001:15(1):25-35
--Legacy S. Treatment of depression in the medically ill. Presentation at October 2001 ABDA Patient/Family Conference, Boston, MA
--Lee S and Bang D. Behçet disease. eMedicine Journal, July 10, 2001;2(7):section6-7
--Sakane T, Takeno M, Suzuki N and Inaba G. Behçet's disease (current concepts). New Engl J Med 1999;341:1284-1291
--Kaklamani VG and Kaklamanis PG. Treatment of Behçet's disease-an update. Semin Arthritis Rheum 2001 Apr;30(5):299-312
--Physician's Drug Handbook. 9th Edition. Springhouse, PA; copyright 2001 by Springhouse Corporation
--Spratto G and Woods A. PDR Nurse's Drug Handbook, 2002 Edition. Medical Economics Company, NJ, copyright 2002 by Delmar
--Suda H. [Low-dose weekly methotrexate therapy for progressive neuro-Behcet's disease]. Nihon Rinsho Meneki Gakkai Kaishi. 1999 Feb;22(1):13-22. Japanese
--Rosenberg R. "Delivering treatment that may be visionary." Boston Globe, June 6, 2001, "Business" section

Drug assistance programs and information for patients meeting financial requirements

Institute Fulfillment Center

PO Box 210
Dallas, PA 18612-0210
www.institute-dc.org

The Institute Fulfillment Center offers two booklets for sale:

1) Free and Low-Cost Prescription Drugs ($5)

Many drug companies offer reduced-price or free prescriptions to patients who meet financial requirements. This booklet lists 78 drug assistance programs and 1100 drugs that are covered, including Remicade (infliximab), Enbrel (etanercept), Methotrexate, Vioxx (rofecoxib), Prilosec, and Zantac . Booklet is 32 pages, and costs $5 by first-class mail with shipping included; $4 for immediate PDF download if paid by credit card online: go to www.institute-dc.org to place the PDF order.

2) Free and Low-Cost Medical Care ($5)

Booklet gives a comprehensive list of facilities that are required to provide free and low-cost medical care under the Hill-Burton Medical Act. Categories include hospital, outpatient and nursing care facilities. Over 700 listings arranged by state; 59 pages, costs $5 (including shipping).

Please allow 1-2 weeks for delivery.

The Medicine Program

For a low fee, this group will provide applications for pharmaceutical assistance programs for specific medications. For more information, go to www.the medicineprogram.com, or call 573-996-7300.

CHAPTER 3

Is it really Behçet's? Or is it Lupus? Or MS, or Crohn's or Lyme...

A diagnosis of Behçet's disease can be a difficult one for patients to receive - and a difficult diagnosis for health care providers to make. Because there is no definitive diagnostic test, months or years may pass before enough major symptoms emerge to point specialists in the right direction. This problem is compounded by the fact that many Behçet's-like symptoms can also appear in other diseases besides BD. The line between illnesses is especially blurred in early stages of the disease, when symptoms may be vague. Illnesses that can initially be confused with BD include lupus (systemic lupus erythematosus or SLE), multiple sclerosis (MS), Crohn's disease, Lyme disease, Reiter's syndrome and Stevens-Johnson syndrome.[19] Rogers (2000) has added to the list by including erythema multiforme, mucous membrane pemphigoid, and the vulvovaginal-gingival form of erosive lichen planus, all of which he has placed under the heading "pseudo-Behçet's disease."[25] BD patients may also receive an unfortunate (and untested) diagnosis of herpes or other sexually transmitted disease, simply due to the presence of genital ulcerations.

It is possible for a Behçet's case to "overlap" with another disease. In other words, some patients may have one or more autoimmune-type illnesses occurring simultaneously, in addition to Behcet's.[5]

The basic symptoms of SLE, MS, Crohn's, Lyme disease, and Reiter's syndrome are described below. Please see your health care provider if you have specific questions about your own symptoms, based on anything that you read in this chapter.

SLE (systemic lupus erythematosus):

According to the Lupus Foundation of America (1300 Piccard Dr, Ste 200, Rockville, MD 20850-4303; 1-800-558-0121), the following symptoms occur most frequently in lupus:[29]

Achy joints (arthralgia)	95% of cases
Unexplained fever >100F (38C)	90%
Arthritis (swollen joints)	90%
Prolonged or extreme fatigue	81%
Skin rashes	74%
Anemia	71%
Kidney inflammation (nephritis)	50%
Chest pain when breathing deeply (pleurisy)	45%

Butterfly-shaped rash across cheeks & nose	42%
Sun or light sensitivity (photosensitivity)	30%
Hair loss	27%
Abnormal blood clotting problems	20%
Raynaud's phenomenon (fingers and/or toes turn white or blue in the cold)	17%
Seizures	15%
Mouth or nose ulcers	12%

According to the NIH,[1] lupus-related **kidney inflammation** may not be painful, but may cause swelling in the hands, feet or legs.

Involvement of the **central nervous system (CNS)** may cause headaches, dizziness, memory disturbances, vision problems [visual blurring or loss of some vision[8]], stroke, or changes in behavior. However, these symptoms may also be caused by some medications, or by emotional stress.

Blood vessels may become inflamed [vasculitis]. There may be an increased risk of anemia, blood clots, leukopenia [a decrease in the number of white blood cells] or thrombocytopenia [a decrease in the number of platelets in the blood].

The **heart** may experience pericarditis [inflammation of the lining of the heart], myocarditis [inflammation of the heart muscle] or coronary artery disease. These heart problems can occur in 20-30% of people with lupus.

Diagnosis of SLE:

An SLE diagnosis is based on experiencing four or more of the following 11 criteria, which can appear at the same time, or over a period of time.[7]

1) Malar (butterfly) rash across cheeks and nose
2) Discoid rash: a scaly, red, disc-shaped raised rash, usually on the face, neck, scalp, ears, chest, or arms.
3) Photosensitivity: a rash or severe burn caused by unusual sensitivity to sunlight
4) Oral ulcers
5) Arthritis
6) Pleuritis or pericarditis
7) Kidney involvement (proteinuria > 0.5 grams/day or > 3+ if quantitation not performed, OR cellular casts)
8) Central nervous system involvement (seizures in the absence of "offending" drugs or metabolic disorders, OR psychosis in the absence of drugs or metabolic disorders)
9) Blood disorders (hemolytic anemia, OR leukopenia, OR lymphohenia OR thrombocytopenia)
10) Immunologic abnormalities (positive LE cell test OR anti-DNA OR anti-Sm OR false-positive syphilis test)
11) Positive antinuclear antibody (ANA)

Multiple Sclerosis (MS):

Multiple sclerosis is a disease where the nerves of the eye, brain, and spinal cord lose patches of myelin. Myelin surrounds nerve fibers in the body, and helps to transmit electrical impulses quickly and accurately. When the myelin sheath surrounding a nerve fiber (axon) is damaged or destroyed, it can cause a variety of medical problems depending on the location of the damage.

MS usually appears in people who are 20 to 40 years old, and occurs in women more often than it does in men. There are approximately 350,000 people who are currently diagnosed with multiple sclerosis in the US.[9] Some symptoms of MS are similar to those found in cases of neuro-Behçet's, which can make a diagnosis especially difficult.

Possible Symptoms of Multiple Sclerosis [10,11]

Fatigue

Tingling, numbness, or other abnormal sensations in the arms, legs, trunk or face

Difficulty in walking or maintaining balance

Visual difficulties: blurred or double vision, partial blindness, loss of vision from optic neuritis [inflammation of the optic nerve]

Weakness or clumsiness

Dizziness or vertigo

Tremor(s)

Slurred speech

Problems with bladder or bowel control, or constipation

Sexual dysfunction: difficulty in reaching orgasm (men and women), impotence, lack of sensation

Sudden paralysis, as might occur in a stroke

Headaches

Seizures

Problems with speech and/or swallowing [dysphagia]

A report on MS diagnosis was released in July 2001 (McDonald et al) : ***Recommended Diagnostic Criteria for Multiple Sclerosis: Guidelines from the International Panel on the Diagnosis of Multiple Sclerosis***. It can be found in *Annals of Neurology*; 50(1): 121-127. The authors stress the need for all tests to be conducted using state-of-the-art technology, with results that are interpreted by experts in the field.

The panel suggested three test results to aid in the diagnosis of MS,[12] in addition to the physician's observation of patients' clinical signs and symptoms:

MRI Criteria for Brain Abnormality in MS

Three out of four of the following:

1) One gadolinium-enhancing lesion, or nine T2-hyperintense intense lesions if there is no gadolinium enhancing lesion.
2) At least one infratentorial lesion
3) At least one juxtacortical lesion
4) At least three periventricular lesions

CSF Analysis in MS

1) The presence of oligoclonal IgG bands different from any such bands in serum, and/or the presence of an elevated IgG index.

71

2) Lymphocytic pleocytosis should be less than 50/mm.

VEP (Visual Evoked Potentials) in MS

An abnormal VEP, typical of MS, is defined as "delayed, but with a well-preserved wave form." Other types of evoked potential testing were not significant for an MS diagnosis.

Various criteria are used by the authors to distinguish between the newly-suggested classes of MS ("MS", "possible MS", or "not MS", instead of the old terminology - "probable MS" and "clinically definite"). There are also well-defined criteria for the number of attacks necessary for diagnosis, as well as the amount of time that passes between attacks. Interested readers are advised to obtain a full copy of the report, due to the obvious diagnostic complexities involved.

One could ask if there are any other research results that could help distinguish between MS and neuro-Behcet's. Rovaris et al (2000) found that spinal cord hyperintense lesions were found on the MRIs of nine out of ten MS patients, but not on the MRIs of any other patient in the study. Behcet's and lupus patients were included in the testing. These spinal cord lesions were found whether or not there were lesions in the brain, and suggests the use of cervical cord MRI to aid in differential diagnosis.[13] And finally, Coban et al (1999) found that the MRIs of patients with an acute attack of neuro-BD showed lesions in the brain stem and/or basal ganglia. However, the MRIs of patients with chronic neuro-BD were hard to distinguish from those of MS patients - in fact, 60% of the chronic NBD cases in the study were misdiagnosed as MS, based solely on their imaging results.[14]

Crohn's Disease

Crohn's disease (CD) has many symptoms similar to the gastrointestinal complications of Behcet's disease. According to the Crohn's and Colitis Foundation of America, Crohn's is a form of inflammatory bowel disease that can cause diarrhea, loss of appetite, abdominal pain, cramping, malabsorption of nutrients, fever, nausea/vomiting, constipation, and weight loss. Similar GI problems are experienced by 10-50% of Behcet's patients.[15,18] Both Behçet's and Crohn's patients may also experience inflammation and pain in the lower right abdominal area, along with abdominal distention [swelling].[22,24]

There are several non-GI-related health problems associated with Crohn's:[16,17]

Non-GI complications of Crohn's disease

Visual complications: uveitis, episcleritis [inflammation of the outer coating of the eye], keratopathy [a corneal abnormality], dry eyes, possible inflammation of other eye structures

Skin lesions: erythema nodosum, pyoderma gangrenosum, and aphthous ulcers

Arthritis

Anemia

Kidney and uric acid stones
Frequent urinary tract infections as a result of fistula formation -
    abnormal connections between inflamed parts of the
    bowel and other areas such as the bladder
Amyloidosis
Glomerulonephritis

In addition, Turner (1992) has described primary and secondary
genital (vulvar) lesions that can occur in Crohn's patients. These
lesions include noncaseating granulomas, as well as non-specific
reactions such as erythema nodosum-like lesions, aphthae, and
pyoderma gangrenosum.[26]
    Crohn's disease creates ileitis [inflammation of the ileum — the
lower part of the small intestine] approximately 35% of the time,
inflammation in the ileum and colon combined (ileocolitis) 45% of the
time, and affects the colon alone in 20% of cases.[22] The main areas of
involvement in BD are the terminal ileum and cecum, as well as the
esophagus and - occasionally - the stomach.[18] However, Crohn's disease,
like Behçet's, has the potential to occur anywhere in the digestive tract,
from the mouth to the anus.[20]
    One of the common imaging characteristics of Crohn's is a
distinct "cobblestone" appearance of the affected bowel.[18] The imaging
hallmarks of GI-Behçet's are the presence of deep, penetrating or
punched-out ulcers, uneven thickening of the bowel wall, and the absence
of granulomas (although granulomas are also absent in up to 50% of
Crohn's patients). The GI ulcers may create a high number of complications, such as bowel perforation, fistulas, hemorrhage, and peritonitis.[18]
    There is no specific lab test that can diagnose Crohn's disease;
however, patients may show signs of anemia, abnormally high white
blood cell counts, and low albumin levels.[21] Complicating the diagnostic
picture even further is the fact that some confirmed Behçet's patients
described in the literature "overlap" with inflammatory bowel disease -
in other words, these patients have symptoms of Behçet's, in addition to
health problems commonly found in Crohn's or ulcerative colitis.[23]
    Interested readers should obtain a copy of **Radiologic findings of
Behcet syndrome involving the gastrointestinal tract**. Radiographics 2001;21:911-924, for more in-depth descriptions of Behçet's GI
involvement. The article also includes 35 excellent CT and barium study
images showing sample lesions in various areas of the GI tract.

Lyme disease

Lyme disease is caused by the bite of an infected deer tick. According to
the CDC,[2] Lyme disease has appeared in 48 states and the District of
Columbia in the US, with 128,000 cases reported since 1982. However,
only ten states account for the majority of cases: some northeast and
Mid-Atlantic states, the upper north-central states, and some areas of
northern California.
    According to the American Lyme Disease Foundation (Mill

Pond Offices, 293 Route 100, Ste. 204, Somers, NY 10589), the following symptoms are common with Lyme disease:[3]

> *Localized early (acute) stage — appears 3-30 days after tick bite*
> Solid red or bull's-eye rash, usually at the site of the tick bite (appears in 89-90% of cases). Has an average diameter of 5-6 inches, lasts for 3-5 weeks, may or may not be warm to the touch, and is usually not painful or itchy. A dark bruise-like appearance is more common on dark-skinned patients.
> Swelling of lymph glands near the tick bite
> Generalized achiness
> Headache
>
> *Early disseminated stage*
> Two or more rashes not at the site of the tick bite
> Migrating pains in the joints/tendons
> Headache
> Stiff, aching neck
> Facial palsy (facial paralysis similar to Bell's palsy)
> Tingling or numbness in the extremities
> Multiple enlarged lymph glands
> Abnormal pulse
> Sore throat
> Changes in vision (may include unusual forms of conjunctivitis, keratitis, optic nerve disease, uveitis, vitreitis, and other types of posterior segment inflammatory disease)[4]
> Fever of 100 to 102 F
> Severe fatigue
>
> *Late stage (may occur weeks, months or even years after a tick bite)*
> Arthritis (pain/swelling) of one or two large joints
> Disabling neurological disorders (disorientation; confusion; dizziness; short-term memory loss; inability to concentrate, finish sentences or follow conversations; mental "fog")
> Numbness in arms/hands or legs/feet
> Severe headaches
> Cardiac abnormalities

Reiter's Syndrome (aka Reactive Arthritis)

Reiter's syndrome is referred to as "reactive arthritis" because it causes joints to become inflamed in reaction to an infection elsewhere in the body. The first symptoms of reactive arthritis usually appear 2-4 weeks after either a gastrointestinal infection, or infection with a sexually transmitted disease. Typical symptoms include: [27,28]

> Nongonococcal urethritis [urinary tract infection] which usually appears first, possibly accompanied by a vaginal discharge, or inflammation of the cervix or vagina. Men may also experience an inflamed prostate gland and/or a discharge from the penis.
> Conjunctivitis, and/or anterior uveitis with redness, pain and

sensitivity to light; may appear near in time to the urinary tract infection.

Asymmetrical joint pain in the knees, ankles and/or feet is most common, although other areas may be affected, such as the spine. Joints may be swollen, warm and painful.

Small, shallow, painless sores may appear on the tongue, on the roof of the mouth, and/or the end of the penis.

A hard, raised rash can occur, usually on the soles of the feet and/or the palms.

Common laboratory findings in Reiter's syndrome can include anemia, increased white blood cell counts, and an elevated sed rate. In addition, approximately 2/3 of Caucasian Reiter's patients exhibit HLA-B27.

Reactive arthritis may last anywhere from 3-12 months; however, a small percentage of patients may experience continual relapses.

References

(1) National Institutes of Health; http://www.nih.gov/niams/healthinfo/slehandout/symptoms.html, July 2001

(2) Centers for Disease Control and Prevention; http://www.cdc.gov/ncidod/dvbid/lyme/epi.htm, July 2001

(3) American Lyme Disease Foundation; http://www.aldf.com/templates/Lyme.cfm, July 2001

(4) Zaidman GW. The ocular manifestations of Lyme disease. Int Ophthalmol Clin 1997 Spring;37(2):13-28

(5) Rechichi CF. Psoriatic arthritis or overlap syndrome. Ophthalmologica. 1997;211(4):266-7

(6) Horowitz, M and Abrams Brill M. Living with Lupus: A Comprehensive Guide to Understanding and Controlling Lupus While Getting On With Your Life. Plume Books, NY, c.1994, p 67

(7) Klippel J (ed). "Criteria for the Classification of Systemic Lupus Erythematosus" in Primer on the Rheumatic Diseases, 11th Ed. Arthritis Foundation, GA, c.1997, p 462

(8) Horowitz, M and Abrams Brill M. Living with Lupus: A Comprehensive Guide to Understanding and Controlling Lupus While Getting On With Your Life. Plume Books, NY, c.1994, p 73

(9) Berkow, R (ed). The Merck Manual of Medical Information, Home Edition. Pub by Merck Research Laboratories, NJ, c. 1997;p.318-9

(10) Berkow, R (ed). The Merck Manual of Medical Information, Home Edition. Pub by Merck Research Laboratories, NJ, c. 1997;p.320

(11) National Multiple Sclerosis Society, http://www.nationalmssociety.org/Sourcebook-Symptoms.asp, August 2001

(12) McDonald WI et al. Recommended Diagnostic Criteria for Multiple Sclerosis: Guidelines from the International Panel on the Diagnosis of Multiple Sclerosis. Annals of Neurology. July 200; 50(1):121-127

(13) Rovaris M, Viti B, Ciboddo G et al. Cervical cord magnetic resonance imaging findings in systemic immune-mediated diseases. J Neurol Sci 2000 Jun 15;176(2):128-30

(14) Coban O et al. Mased assessment of MRI findings: is it possible to differentiate neuro-Behcet's disease from other central nervous system diseases?

Neuroradiology 1999 Apr;41(4):255-60. Erratum in Neuroradiology 1999 Jul;41(7):550

(15) Lee S et al. Behcet's Disease: A Guide to its Clinical Understanding, Textbook and Atlas. Springer Verlag, 2001, p41

(16) Howard D, Greenwald B, Kaminstein D, and Bonheim N, Zwas F, El Serag H. Sections outlining Crohn's complications. Crohn's and Colitis Foundation of America, http://www.ccfa.org/medcentral/library/comp

(17) Lane K (ed). The Merck Manual of Diagnosis and Therapy, Seventeenth (Centennial) Edition, Crohn's disease, p302-5

(18) Chung SY, Ha HK et al. Radiologic findings of Behcet syndrome involving the gastrointestinal tract. Radiographics. 2001;21:911-924

(19) Lane K (ed). The Merck Manual of Diagnosis and Therapy, Seventeenth (Centennial) Edition, c.1999, Behçet's Disease, p425.

(20) Berkow, R (ed). The Merck Manual of Medical Information, Home Edition. Pub by Merck Research Laboratories, NJ, c. 1997;p.528

(21) Berkow, R (ed). The Merck Manual of Medical Information, Home Edition. Pub by Merck Research Laboratories, NJ, c. 1997;p.529

(22) Lane K (ed). The Merck Manual of Diagnosis and Therapy, Seventeenth (Centennial) Edition, c.1999, Behçet's Disease, p.303

(23) Plotkin, Calabro and O'Duffy (eds.). Behçet's Disease: A Contemporary Synopsis. Futura Publishing, c 1988. In Plotkin, Miscellaneous Clinical Manifestations II: Gastrointestinal Features, p250

(24) Plotkin, Calabro and O'Duffy (eds.). Behçet's Disease: A Contemporary Synopsis. Futura Publishing, c 1988. In Plotkin, Miscellaneous Clinical Manifestations II: Gastrointestinal Features, p240

(25) Rogers III R. PseudoBehcet's disease: challenging diagnostic dilemmas. Yonsei Med J 2000:41(3) Suppl, p11 (26) Turner M. Vulvar manifestations of systemic diseases. Dermatology Clinics 1992:10(2), 445-458

(27) Berkow, R (ed). The Merck Manual of Medical Information, Home Edition. Pub by Merck Research Laboratories, NJ, c. 1997;p.241

(28) Arnett FC. Reactive arthritis (Reiter's syndrome) and enteropathic arthritis. In Primer on the Rheumatic Diseases, c.1997, Arthritis Foundation, GA;p.184-7

CHAPTER 4

Pregnancy, Postpartum, and Behçet's Disease

The following excerpt appeared in **Rheumatic Disease Clinics of North America** in 1989, and is reprinted with the permission of W B Saunders Co. More recent medical study results on pregnancy and Behçet's disease appear after the article.

Behçet's Disease and Pregnancy
Gary L. Klipple and Kathryn K. Riordan

The effect of pregnancy on the activity of Behçet's disease is unclear and may be variable. In convincing individual cases, definite pregnancy-associated remissions and flares of disease are described.[4,7,9,10,12] Larson and Baum describe a 32-year-old woman with prednisone-responsive Behçet's disease manifested by oral and genital ulcers, arthritis and painful acneiform skin lesions, which resolved entirely without medications during gestation [pregnancy], only to relapse several days postpartum [after birth].[7] In the review by Chajek and Fainaru, a woman from Iraq with persistent Behçet's disease manifested by oral and genital ulcerations, arthritis, fever, erythema nodosum, and chorioretinitis is presented, who was resistant to therapy, and develops neurologic and phlebitic [vein inflammation] complications. In 20 years of observation, the only remissions were during her two pregnancies.[1]

Conversely, several reports document relapses during pregnancy, primarily with mucocutaneous manifestations. [6,9] Gestation was consistently associated with severe and prolonged exacerbations of arthritis and mucosal ulcers in a woman reported from Saudi Arabia, who had 10 children. Disease manifestations in this individual became quiescent [quiet] after menopause.[9] Farrag et al describe a gravid [pregnant] female with one prior attack of oral and genital ulcers, who developed severe genital ulceration during week 32 of pregnancy. Postpartum [after delivery], she responded well to a short course of prednisolone without subsequent recurrence of disease during a 1-year follow-up.[3] In another case, a 28-year-old woman with previously mild and undiagnosed manifestations of Behçet's disease developed an exacerbation [flare-up] of oral and genital ulcers and arthritis at 21 weeks of gestation, and iridocyclitis at 25 weeks. Postpartum chronic uveitis with visual loss occurred despite chronic prednisone therapy.[6] In a letter, Hamza et al reviewed their experience with 21 pregnancies in eight women with Behçet's disease diagnosed by at least three major criteria. A remission unrelated to therapy was noted in twelve pregnancies, and an exacerbation in nine despite administration of prednisone at 10 to 15 mg per day. Exacerbations usually consisted of painful genital ulcerations, erythema nodosum, and buccal aphthoses [mouth ulcers]. The individual patient responses were generally not consistent, varying from one pregnancy to another, although one woman experienced a relapse with each of four pregnancies.[5]

Although the number of case reports on which to base an opinion is limited, **Behçet's disease seems to have little effect on fetal outcome** *[emphasis by JZ]*. Review of this literature indicates that even in the setting of active disease and/or treatment with corticosteroids, spontaneous abortions and congenital abnormalities are not reported.[3,4,6,7,12] However, transient [temporary] and presumably transplacentally-acquired Behçet's disease has been observed in the neonate [newborn].[2,8] Lewis and Priestly report on a full-term female infant born to a 33-year-old woman with an eight-year history of Behçet's disease. At birth, a few small pustulonecrotic skin lesions were noted. At eight days, multiple severe oral ulcers and pustulonecrotic skin lesions on the hands and feet, with periungual [around the nail] ulcerations developed. A pathergy reaction occurred at venipuncture [injection] sites. New lesions occurred for up to five weeks, with healing complete at eight weeks, leaving residual scars. Intravenous antibiotics and acyclovir were of no benefit. The authors recommend early consideration of corticosteroid treatment of this entity.[8]

Since fetal outcome is generally good in Behçet's syndrome, disease manifestations are not consistently aggravated, and major complications such as CNS or vascular disease are uncommon, the management of pregnant Behçet's patients is aimed at control of active manifestations with minimal risk to the developing fetus. Potentially teratogenic [causing fetal deformity] **medications** including cyclophosphamide [Cytoxan], chlorambucil [Leukeran], thalidomide, colchicine, and levamisole, should be discontinued before conception. Treatment of active disease with topical preparations, or occasionally local injections of corticosteroids, are reasonable alternatives to systemic therapy.[11] When required, prednisone or prednisolone are the drugs of choice to control major systemic manifestations of Behçet's disease during gestation. A role for therapeutic abortion, early induction of labor, or caesarean section have not been defined.

Footnotes to WB Saunders article (above)
1) Chajek T, Fainaru M. Behçet's disease. Report of 41 cases and review of the literature. Medicine 1975;54:179-96
2) Fam Ag, Siminovitch KA, Carette S, et al. Neonatal Behçet's syndrome in an infant of a mother with the disease. Ann Rheum Dis 1981;40:509-12
3) Farrag OA, Al-Suleiman SA, Bella H, et al. Behcet disease during pregnancy. Aust NZ J Obstet Gynaecol 1987;27:161-163
4) Ferraro G, Lomeo C, Mascarelli G, et al. A case of pregnancy in a patient

suffering from Behçet's syndrome. Immunologic aspects. Acta Eur Fertil 1984;15:67-72

5) Hamza M, Elleuch M, Zrib A. Behçet's disease and pregnancy. Ann Rheum Dis 1988;47:350

6) Hurt WG, Cooke CL, Jordan WP, et al. Behçet's syndrome associated with pregnancy. Obstet Gynecol 1979;53:31A-33S

7) Larsson L-G, Baum J. Behçet's syndrome in pregnancy and after the delivery. J Rheumatol 1987;14:183

8) Lewis MA, Priestley BL. Transient neonatal Behçet's disease. Arch Dis Child 1986;61:805-806

9) Madkour M, Kudwah A. Behçet's disease. Br Med J1978;ii:1786

10) Plouvier B, Devulder B. Behçet's disease. Br Med J 1979;I:690

11) Shimizu T, Ehrlich GE, Inaba G, et al. Behcet disease (Behcet syndrome). Sem Arthritis Rheum 1979;8:223-260

12) Suchenwirth RMA: Beitrag zum Problem Morbus Behcet and Nervensystem. 10 jahrige Verlaufsbeobachtung mit Schwangerschafte/Literaturubersicht. Fortschr Neurol Psychiatr 1984;52:41-7

Twelve years after the above article was published, we are not much closer to understanding which patients will have flare-ups of Behçet's symptoms during pregnancy, and which ones will go into a pregnancy-inspired remission. However, some additional articles have been published on the subject since that time.

One Turkish study (Gul, 2000) followed sixteen Behçet's patients before, during, and after pregnancy.[1] **Symptom flare-ups** occurred during pregnancy for nine of the sixteen women, with the noted problems being frequent genital ulcers, major oral ulcers, papulopustular skin lesions, and erythema nodosum. Flare-ups occurred after delivery for three of the women, two of whom had been in remission before and during pregnancy. These women experienced frequent oral ulcers after delivery, along with genital ulcers, erythema nodosum and uveitis. What about remission of symptoms? Seven women (44%) of the original sixteen patients experienced a **total remission [absence] of symptoms** during their pregnancies. All sixteen pregnancies in the study resulted in **normal deliveries** of healthy babies.

Bang, Chun et al published a study in 1997[2] that followed twenty-seven Behçet's patients who were pregnant. Approximately 67% of the women had a worsening of their symptoms during pregnancy, while 33% improved during the same time period. If Behçet's-related health problems occurred, they showed up most often during the **first trimester**. Patients whose health improved during pregnancy tended to be the ones whose Behçet's flare-ups regularly got worse immediately before or during their **menstrual periods**.

Marsal et al (1997) performed a study looking at 61 pregnancies occurring in 23 women with Behçet's disease.[3] They compared these women with two other groups: a group of 20 healthy women with 61 total pregnancies between them, and a group of 30 women with recurrent oral ulcers, who had a total of 83 pregnancies between them. The researchers found that there was no difference in the rate of pregnancy complications between the groups, and there was **no relationship between Behçet's disease and the occurrence of congenital problems** [problems present at birth]. In contrast to the other reports mentioned above, only two patients in this study had Behçet's-related symptom flare-ups during their pregnancies - a scant 9%, compared to the unfortunate 67% of women included in the Bang study in 1997.

Two studies have specifically addressed the relationship between pregnancy and Behçet's-induced **visual problems**. Taguchi et al (1999) described a Behçet's patient whose constant uveitis inflammations slowed down markedly during her pregnancy, even though she was removed from all medications.[4] Her uveitis has been in almost complete remission since delivery. In addition, in a presentation at the 1999 ABDA Conference, a neuro-ophthalmologist described possible connections between pregnancy and uveitis flare-ups in Behçet's patients. In general, pregnancy was associated with stability of vision. However, the following conclusions were also drawn:[5]

1) Women who experienced Behçet's-related eye inflammations during pregnancy tended to get their flare-ups during the first trimester. In the second trimester, problems tended to level off, and then to stabilize during the third trimester.

2) Anterior uveitis, if it appeared at all, occurred mostly in the first trimester.

3) If visual problems were going to appear after delivery, it was usually during the first six weeks postpartum.

4) Patients who experienced uveitis during their pregnancies had the highest risk of recurrences following delivery.

Fibromyalgia (FM) is a subject that is rarely mentioned in relation to Behçet's patients, let alone pregnant Behçet's patients. Fibromyalgia causes aches, pain and stiffness in muscles, tendons and ligaments, and is identified by pain at specific "trigger points" on parts of the body. Ostensen et al (1997) published a study looking at the relationship of fibromyalgia symptoms to pregnant patients in general.[6] The subject of Behçet's was not mentioned. Twenty-six fibromyalgic women with a total of forty pregnancies were included in this study. The researchers found that all of the women, except one, had an increase in their fibromyalgia symptoms during pregnancy, with the last trimester providing the worst FM-related problems. In thirty-three of the forty pregnancies, patients also experienced a worsening of their symptoms during the six months following delivery. In addition, postpartum depression and anxiety increased. Prior to becoming pregnant, 72% of the patients enrolled in this study usually had a worsening of their FM symptoms before menstruation.

There has been one official report in the literature of Behçet's disease associated with **intrauterine growth restriction (IUGR)**, where a fetus is abnormally small in development: at or below the tenth percentile in weight while in the uterus. IUGR has been described by Johnson (1997) as an uncommon condition that affects only 3-7% of *all* pregnancies, and can be caused by decreased blood flow between the uterus and placenta.[8] Guzelian (1997) wrote of a 27-year old woman who experienced several Behçet's-related flare-ups of oral and genital ulcers throughout her pregnancy, and delivered a severely growth-restricted baby at 36 1/2 weeks, following evidence of fetal distress.[9] He suggests that pregnancies complicated by Behçet's disease be followed closely for such possible high-risk complications. *[As an aside, IUGR occurred during this writer's first pregnancy, when Behçet's disease was suspected but not yet diagnosed. Fetal growth stopped at 30 weeks, and fetal movement slowed drastically. Delivery was by C-section at 37 weeks, following evidence of fetal distress. After a rocky start, this son is now thirteen years old, healthy, and above the growth charts in height.]*

Bergant et al (2000) mentioned the case of a 28-year-old pregnant woman of Mediterranean heritage, whose child was delivered by C-section.[7] Her previous medical history included many features common to Behçet's disease, although her pregnancy was free of health problems. Nine days after delivery, she developed a high fever with inflammation of both nipples, leading to the formation of deep ulcers on her nipples. This painful complication forced her to stop breastfeeding. The ulcers were eventually healed with topical and systemic treatments. Bergant suggested that the ulcerations formed because of the "mechanical irritation" involved in breastfeeding.

The following excerpt may assist women in wishing to know what drugs they may take during their pregnancies, and while breastfeeding.

From *The Effects of Immunosuppressive and Anti-inflammatory Medications on Fertility, Pregnancy, and Lactation:*[10]

"Many rheumatic diseases affect women of childbearing age, and the medications used to treat these diseases may affect conception, pregnancy, fetal development, and lactation. Physicians who care for these women need to be aware of the potential adverse effects of these medications, and which medications can be used safely prior to conception and during pregnancy and lactation. Although reviews of individual classes of medications are available, there is no practical and comprehensive review that summarizes all of this information, and includes anticoagulant drugs and two recently approved drugs for rheumatoid arthritis. Women who take cytotoxic drugs should be informed of the risks of impaired fertility and congenital malformations, and must use effective methods of contraception. During pregnancy, non-steroidal anti-inflammatory agents [NSAIDS] may be used until the last 6 weeks, and low to moderate doses of corticosteroids are safe throughout pregnancy. Among the disease-modifying agents, sulfasalazine [Azulfidine] and hydroxychloroquine [Plaquenil] treatment may be maintained. Cytotoxic drugs may be used after the first trimester to treat life-threatening disease. During lactation, prednisone, sulfasalazine and hydroxychloroquine may be used cautiously. Women using heparin for treatment of antiphospholipid antibody syndrome should take measures to prevent bone loss. Men taking methotrexate, sulfasalazine, cyclosporine, azathioprine [Imuran], or leflunomide should be apprised of the possibilities of infertility and teratogenicity."

*[JZ: Women who are planning a pregnancy or caring for small children may be interested in visiting the following website: www.revma.org This is the internet home of the **Center for Mothers with Rheumatic Disease**, which is located in Norway. Their mailing address is: Center for Mothers with Rheumatic Disease, Department of Rheumatology, University Hospital of Trondheim, N-7006 Trondheim, Norway.]*

References
1) Gul U, Arch Dermatol 2000;Aug;136(8):1063-4
2) Bang D, Chun YS et al. The influence of pregnancy on Behçet's Disease; Yonsei Med J Dec;38(6):437-43
3) Marsal et al. Behçet's disease and pregnancy relationship study; Br J Rheumatol;1997 Feb;36(2):234-8
4) Taguchi C et al. A report of two cases suggesting positive influence of pregnancy on uveitis activity; Nippon Ganka Gakkai Zasshi 1999 Jan;103(1):66-71
5) Chavis P. Presentation of unpublished conclusions; American Behçet's Disease Association conference, September 1999, Nashville, TN
6) Ostensen M et al. The effect of reproductive events and alterations of sex hormone levels on the symptoms of fibromyalgia; Scand J Rheumatol 1997;26(5):355-60
7) Bergant A et al. Bilateral nipple ulcers in a breastfeeding woman: a manifestation of Behçet's disease; Brit J Obs Gyn; October 2000, Vol 107;1320-1322
8) Johnson MJ. Obstetric complications and rheumatic disease. In "Pregnancy and Rheumatic Disease" chapter of Rheumatic Disease Clinics of North America 1997;23(1):175-6
9) Guzelian G, Norton ME. Behçet's syndrome associated with intrauterine growth restriction: a case report and review of the literature. J Perinatol 1997;Jul-Aug;17(4):318-20
10) Janssen N and Genta M. The effects of immunosuppressive and anti-inflammatory medications on fertility, pregnancy, and lactation. Arch Intern Med 2000;160:610-619

CHAPTER 5

Behçet's disease in children

Does Behçet's disease occur in young people? It can and it does, affecting children at any age from newborn through the late teen years. Pediatric cases of BD are "uncommon" according to medical researchers,[1] as the majority of Behçet's cases begin when patients are in their 20s or 30s. However, the amount of literature on the topic of pediatric Behçet's has increased in recent years. As a result, we may see a rise in the number of reported cases of childhood BD, as pediatricians - and parents - become more familiar with the diagnosis.

Behçet's in newborn babies

"Neonatal Behçet's disease" is the appearance of BD symptoms in newborns up to six weeks of age. The symptoms typically appear within one week of birth[2] and usually clear up within two to three months. In four out of the six reported cases of neonatal BD, the mothers were diagnosed with Behçet's prior to pregnancy.[3,4,5,6] In the first case, a newborn boy developed a fever, oral and genital ulcerations, and pustular skin lesions on his face, scalp, and buttocks. The lesions resolved after six weeks, leaving scars in their place. The baby had no further symptoms, although the length of time for medical follow-up was unclear.

In the second situation, a newborn boy developed ulcerations in his mouth and throat, with pustular lesions on his hands and feet. Again, all symptoms disappeared within six weeks, with no apparent relapse.

In the third situation, a newborn girl developed pustular lesions on her hands and feet, along with numerous mouth ulcers. All lesions healed within eight weeks, leaving scar tissue.

In the fourth case, a newborn girl developed blister-like lesions on her scalp, arms and legs; she also had mouth and throat ulcerations in addition to oral and genital sores. Lab tests ruled out herpes as the ulceration source. All lesions healed within three weeks, leaving scars.

Why did these babies develop short-term cases of Behçet's? According to El-Roeiy and Shoenfeld (1985), "[an] important aspect of autoimmune diseases during pregnancy entails the passive transfer of the disease into the fetal compartment."[7] The tentative "transfer vehicle" may be IgG antibodies, according to a report by Stark et al in

1997.[2] While there are several different kinds of antibodies in the immune system, IgG antibodies are the only ones that can cross the placental barrier from the mother to the fetus. In healthy individuals, these antibodies are responsible for providing temporary immunity in newborns for some illnesses during the first few weeks of life. In a woman with Behçet's, the same antibodies that create her health problems may also cross the placenta and cause temporary but similar problems in the newborn. After several weeks, these antibodies (and the infant's resulting medical problems) tend to disappear. According to Stark, "IgG is cleared from the [newborn's] circulation within four months, accounting for the transient nature of the illness."[2] While an infant's Behçet's-related health issues may recede without treatment, Lewis and Priestley (1986) strongly suggest the short-term use of corticosteroids, to eliminate the possibility of disfiguring scars caused by severe ulcerations.[3] This treatment should only be initiated after testing to rule out possible infectious causes for the lesions, such as herpes or staphylococcus.[6]

If a mother's antibodies are responsible for the development of neonatal Behçet's, then alert readers might question why **all** newborns of mothers with Behçet's disease don't develop neonatal BD. It appears that, just as Behçet's in adults currently has no single, identifiable cause, other factors besides antibodies are at work to create this neonatal illness. A genetic pre-disposition may be necessary, in addition to other possible environmental or infectious triggers.

Only one research report was found that showed an unfortunate escalation of Behçet's symptoms during, and beyond, the neonatal stage. Chong et al (1988) described a Pakistani brother and sister who developed recurrent mouth ulcers and unremitting diarrhea during the first few weeks following birth; treatment with oral prednisolone and sulphasalazine did not eliminate these problems. Continued diarrhea, with extensive inflammation and ulcerations, eventually required almost total removal of the colon in each child. Several years later, the children still have occasional bloody diarrhea, but no other Behçet's symptoms.[8]

We leave this subject with one last, curious, case of neonatal BD. Stark et al (1997) described a woman whose very first experience with Behçet's-type symptoms occurred during her second pregnancy, when she developed oral and genital ulcers and a sore throat in the second trimester.[2] Once these problems healed, the rest of her pregnancy was uneventful. However, five days after delivery, her newborn son developed bloody diarrhea, along with severe mouth and genital ulcerations and skin lesions. On the twenty-second day after birth, her baby's condition began to worsen, with a cough, fever, and an elevated white blood cell count. At six weeks, he went into respiratory arrest and was temporarily placed on a ventilator. Amazingly, at the age of eight weeks, the infant had completely recovered due to the administration of IV and oral steroids.

Stark notes that there are two unusual features found in this case: the mother's Behçet's-related symptoms returned when the baby was 24 days old, at a time when her child's health problems began to worsen; and the fact that the mother had never shown any BD symptoms until her pregnancy, which is not typical in the world of Behçet's.

As a result, Stark raises an interesting hypothesis: "Although the most likely course of events is that the mother developed Behçet's disease in pregnancy and transmitted it by an immune mechanism to the infant during pregnancy, it is also conceivable that Behçet's disease was transmitted to the mother from the affected fetus. Vertical transmission from infant to mother could explain the relatively minor symptoms in the mother compared to the infant....We postulate that disease in both infant and mother may have been exacerbated postpartum by an unidentified infectious agent. This could explain why the infant became so unwell late in the course of the transient neonatal disease when, in fact, levels of immunoglobulins should be falling."[2]

Behçet's in children

Many parents are unsure what to expect in a child with Behçet's disease. Will certain symptoms occur more frequently than others? Are there differences between the health problems that children experience, and the medical issues of adults with Behçet's? What kinds of medications can be used to help these younger members of the BD community? One would hope that the answers to these questions would be straightforward, and treatments easily implemented. However, pediatric Behçet's is far from being completely understood. Here are a few examples of statements from different medical journals, showing some conflicting research results:

> "Behçet's disease in children is similar to the disease in adults."[9]

> "The clinical course of Behçet's disease in children is less severe than in adults."[10]

> "Our results point to a similar systemic expression of BD in children and adults; however, the disease seems to run a less severe course in children."[11]

> "The clinical progress of Behçet's disease in the pediatric age group was similar to that found in adult disease."[12]

> "Severe Behçet's disease in children and juveniles shows no age or sex [preference], but leads to an earlier recurrence and more severe systemic signs."[13]

And here are some examples of symptoms reported in medical journal articles on pediatric Behçet's patients. Some statements might appear to conflict with each other; however, these statements may instead be showing how childhood BD manifests itself in different parts of the world.

> "According to the literature, pediatric Behçet's disease is characterized by a **low incidence of ocular lesions** and a **high incidence of intestinal involvement**."[14]

85

"**Chronic episodic fever** of unknown origin [in children] is characterized by fever lasting for a few days to a few weeks, followed by a fever-free interval and a sense of well-being. The main causes are familial Mediterranean fever...[etc, and] Behcet disease...."[18]

"**Ocular involvement in childhood may be very severe**. Young males, as adult males, showed an earlier onset of the disease and a worse ocular prognosis."[15]

"Recent surveys of patients have outlined peculiar features in this age group such as recurrent attacks of **fever and abdominal pain**. Considered to be uncommon in childhood, **uveitis** have [sic] a very severe course."[16]

"Children with BD had significantly **[fewer] genital ulcers, [fewer] vascular thromboses** and **more non-specific gastrointestinal symptoms** [than adults], as well as **central nervous system involvement and arthralgia**. A relatively high prevalence of uveitis was found in childhood BD."[11]

"The most frequent minor sign [of BD in children] was **arthritis**....The most frequent major sign was **oral ulceration**, appearing in all patients. Other major signs were **genital ulcers, skin lesions and ocular lesions**."[10]

"**Uveitis** was less frequent than in adults but carried a poor prognosis, especially in male patients."[17]

"...the initial symptoms associated with Behçet's disease were **oral aphthous lesions or genital ulcers**. Sixteen [out of 18 subjects] developed ocular symptoms in a later stage...**Posterior uveitis** was the most common [ocular] manifestation."[12]

"**Gastrointestinal signs and symptoms** were more frequent in childhood Behcet disease than in adults, while **ocular complications were less frequent**."[20]

For many parents, the above list of health problems is not only confusing - it can also seem overwhelming. It may be most useful, therefore, to provide an overview of the range of symptoms that have been seen in children with Behçet's, as found in several research studies.

The information in the following table has been compiled from eight studies involving a total of 249 children with Behçet's disease. The studies originated in France,[29] the United Kingdom,[9] Japan,[33] Israel,[11] Korea,[10] Tunisia,[34] Iran,[35] and Turkey.[12] Not all symptoms were discussed in every research study.

Frequency of symptoms reported in 249 pediatric Behçet's cases

Symptom	Percentage of patients	# patients w/symptom
Mouth ulcers*	94% of childhood cases*	233 out of 249 tudied
Genital ulcers	53% (range = 26-82%)	132 / 249
Skin lesions	61% (range = 35-90%)	153 / 249
Joint pains	39% (range = 32-60%)	30 / 77

Arthritis	18% (range = 10-32%)	33 / 188
Headaches	17% (range = 2-37%)	18 / 107
Neurological	14% (range = 10-26%)	19 / 132
GI problems	28% (range = 5-55%)	42 / 148
Eye involvement	36% (range = 20-80%)	60 / 168
Positive pathergy	32% (range = 17-65%)	23 / 71
Perianal ulcers	21% (range = 14-30%)	5 / 24
Intracranial hypertension	16% (range = 11-21%)	7 / 43

mouth ulcers occurred in 100% of children in all studies except Iran

While the above table is useful in a general way, it may also be helpful to list the kinds of health problems reported in the different symptom categories. Unless otherwise indicated by footnotes, all health problems listed below were found within one or more of the eight research studies used to create the above table. **Please note:** the inclusion of items on this list does not mean that every child with Behçet's will eventually develop each of these health problems. They are provided as examples of medical issues that have faced children who have been included in Behçet's research studies. In addition, it is important to remember that some of the problems on this list can also be caused by medical conditions other than Behçet's. It is always best to seek professional medical advice and treatment whenever new or unusual health problems arise.

Health problems reported in children who have been included in Behçet's research studies:

Skin lesions: erythema nodosum [red and painful nodules, usually on the legs]; pseudofolliculitis [according to Kim et al, "folliculitis-like lesions of Behçet's disease are different from other types of folliculitis in that they have less tendency to form pustules on the papules, often spontaneously disappear, and do not respond to antibiotic therapy];[10] papulopustular lesions or rash; leukocytoclastic vasculitis of the skin; necrotic folliculitis; erythema multiforme-like rash [non-itchy dark red rash, usually appearing in rings or disk-shaped patches];[40] external ear ulceration;[40] "various skin rashes that appear and disappear spontaneously;"[41] lymphocytic vasculitis;[31] acneiform nodules [according to Kim et al, they are "different from acne in normal adolescents or adults in that pruritis [itching] and comedone [blackhead] formation are unusual."][10]

Joint pains [arthralgia] or arthritis: pain in the knees, ankles and hip joints; inflammation in the knee, ankle, elbow and hand/finger joints; telalgia [pain in the heel or ankle];[1] "migratory arthralgias" [pain moving from one joint to another];[40] low back pain.[22]

Headaches: may be recurrent, include vomiting, and may be a sign of neurologic problems. According to Vignola et al (2001), "Headache has been regarded as a possible lone clinical manifestation of pediatric neuro-Behçet's, and recent neuroimaging findings in adulthood are in line with this interpretation. In fact, isolated headache, which is observed frequently, is not always taken into right account to define neuro-Behçet's...agreement is still lacking on this issue, and whether headache must be considered a risk factor for developing more serious neurologic involvement in the long term is still debated. Features of headache in this series included...the poor response to common analgesics and NSAIDS."[22] In addition, Vignola found that brain perfusional SPECT helped to spot brain abnormalities in all of the pediatric patients in his study, even when other testing appeared normal.

Neurological problems: meningoencephalitis [inflammation of the brain and surrounding membranes], pseudotumor cerebri [also known as benign intracranial hypertension, which is an increase in pressure around the brain; it may cause headache and optic nerve inflammation], aseptic meningitis [may cause fever, headache, neck pain/ stiffness, decreased level of consciousness], papilledema [inflammation of the optic nerve]; muscle weakness; peripheral neuropathy [pain, tingling and/or numbness in the limbs;[1] seizures; impaired memory / memory loss;[40] cranial nerve palsy [can cause temporary or permanent loss or dysfunction of hearing, balance, vision, smell, swallowing, facial and tongue movement, or eye movements]; hyperreflexia [increased reflexes];[41] hemihypoesthesia [dimished sensation on one side of the body];[31] stroke;[31] optic neuritis;[31] diplopia [double vision].[31]

Gastrointestinal problems: repeated and/or non-specific abdominal pain; bloody or non-bloody diarrhea; colicky abdominal pain; pharyngeal or esophageal stenosis [narrowing of the pharynx or esophagus, possibly related to scar tissue from ulcerations]; GI tract ulcerations [40] [can occur anywhere in the GI tract, from the mouth to the anus]; "the [full] spectrum of gastrointestinal involvement, from minimal irregularity and thickening of the terminal ileum to gross irregularity and deformity of the terminal ileum and cecum."[36]

Pulmonary [lungs]: recurrent pleuritis [inflammation of the membrane surrounding both lungs], pulmonary aneurysm; pleural effusion [fluid in the chest].

Eye involvement: problems may involve one or both eyes: anterior uveitis; posterior uveitis; retinal vasculitis; panuveitis (inflammation of the entire uveal tract, which is the middle vascular layer of the eye); decreased vision; blurred vision;[41] hypopyon [pus in the anterior chamber of the eye]; recurrent conjunctivitis; [40] possible long-term complications including glaucoma, cataracts and optic atrophy; vitreal hemorrhage;[25] keratitis [inflammation of the cornea];[41] iridocyclitis [inflammation of the iris and ciliary body];[41] episcleritis [inflammation of the outermost layer of the membrane surrounding the eyeball];[41] chorioretinitis [inflammation of the choroid and the retina];[41] hyalitis [inflammation of the vitreous];[32] photophobia [intolerance to light].

Psychiatric problems: severe anxiety; personality changes.

**Vascular involvement:** deep or superficial vein thrombosis of the lower limbs; superior sagittal sinus thrombosis; Budd-Chiari syndrome with ascites, hepatomegaly and superior vena cava syndrome; inferior vena cava thrombosis; dural sinus thrombosis; thrombophlebitis; deep vein thrombosis.

**Miscellaneous symptoms:** epididymitis / orchitis [inflammation of one or both testicles]; prolonged or recurring fever of unknown origin;[39] hepatomegaly [liver enlargement];[1] pericarditis [inflammation of the membrane enclosing the heart];[40] myositis [inflammation of muscle tissue, causing pain, swelling and tenderness of the affected area];[40] neutropenia [abnormally small number of neutrophil cells in the blood];[40] splenomegaly [spleen enlargement];[40] kidney involvement with amyloidosis; hematuria [blood in the urine]; thrombocytopenia [abnormal decrease in blood platelet level]; myalgias [tenderness or pain in the muscles];[40] ulcerations of the pharynx.[27]

While this listing can give readers an idea of the potential health problems facing children with Behcet's, it does not necessarily help parents to understand which problems are more serious than others. Krause et al provided a "Severity" overview in their 1999 study,[11] based on an earlier article by Yosipovitch et al in 1995.[43]

Suggested levels of severity in Behçet's disease _(Krause et al, 1999):_

The following problems may be indicators of "mild" Behçet's disease: Oral ulcers; genital ulcers; typical skin lesions (such as erythema nodosum, papulopustular lesions, folliculitis); leukocytoclastic vasculitis; joint pains; recurrent headaches; epididymitis; mild gastrointestinal symptoms such as chronic diarrhea and chronic recurrent colicky abdominal pain; pleuritic pain [caused by inflammation of the membranes surrounding the lungs]; and superficial vein thrombosis.

The following problems may be indicators of "moderate" Behçet's disease: Arthritis; deep vein thrombosis of the legs; anterior uveitis; gastrointestinal bleeding.

The following problems are indicators of "severe" Behçet's disease: Posterior uveitis; panuveitis; retinal vasculitis; arterial thrombosis or aneurysms; major vein (vena cava, hepatic) thrombosis; neuro-Behçet's; bowel perforation.

Conclusions from various researchers regarding some Behçet's symptoms in children:

"**Oral ulceration**, which is the most common initial manifestation [in childhood Behçet's], should not be neglected in children, since it may signal [eventual] Behçet's disease."[10]

"Previous studies have demonstrated a high frequency of **oral ulcers** among family members of patients with BD. We found similar rates of familial aphthosis (recurrent aphthous stomatitis in a close family member) in children and adults."[11]

"**Perianal aphthosis** [ulceration around the anus] is probably particular to Juvenile BD. It occurred in 14% in this study and in 6% in the series of Kone et al, and is very rare in adult BD."[34]

[In a personal comment, persistent/episodic fever, abdominal pain, and "migrating" joint pains are problems that parents mention frequently during personal discussions of their childrens' Behçet's symptoms. Additional information can be found in the stories of three children with Behçet's (8, 12, and 16 years old) in the book, **You Are Not Alone: 15 People with Behçet's** - JZ]

Medications used in the treatment of Behçet's in children

Most of the drugs for children that are listed in this section are also used to help adults who are dealing with BD-related health problems; physicians scale dosages down to help pediatric patients. Parents should consult carefully with their child's doctor(s) when choosing a treatment plan, and discuss all possible side effects in advance. Because there is no "magic pill" to cure Behçet's, there is often an agonizing trade-off during drug selection: which medications will do the most good, with the fewest possible side effects? It is important to know that the medications that work for one child may have little or no effect on the symptoms of another pediatric patient. As a result, it may take several trial-and-error attempts to settle on a dosage and drug schedule that works best for your child. Please note that brand names listed below are meant as examples only, and are not an endorsement of one product over any others.

In a quick review of the literature, the following drugs have been mentioned in the treatment of Behçet's-type symptoms in children (this is only a partial list; many other medications are also available): oral steroids such as prednisone; colchicine; COX-2 inhibitors [Celebrex/Vioxx]; azathioprine [Imuran]; leflunomide [Arava]; hydroxychloroquine [Plaquenil]; sulfasalazine [Azulfidine]; methotrexate [Rheumatrex]; cyclophosphamide [Cytoxan]; cyclosporine [Sandimmune]; mycophenolate mofetil (CellCept); stem-cell transplants; alpha interferon; and thalidomide [Thalomid]. Specific uses for these drugs (as well as other medications) can be found in the chapter on **Treatment** in this book. Additional description is provided below on the following medications: thalidomide, alpha interferon, and fluticasone propionate.

Thalidomide has an especially unpleasant history of causing fetal birth defects, but has made a resurgence in recent years in the treatment of severe ulcerations. According to Kari et al (2001): "Thalidomide provided a useful therapeutic option for severe [pediatric] oral and genital ulceration which was unresponsive to other therapies. Awareness of the danger of axonal neuropathy and teratogenesis [fetal defects] at all times during thalidomide therapy is crucial. A low dose is probably as effective as higher doses."[9] Brik et all (2001) also used thalidomide successfully in treating an 11-month old child with severe oral ulcers, and with GI lesions that were causing diarrhea.[30] However, a journal review of thalidomide's use in pediatric patients (Bessmertny and Pham, 2002) cautions that, in almost all cases, symptoms recur as soon as the drug is discontinued.[51] The authors suggest that thalidomide only be used in children "as a last resort when all other therapies fail, preferably in male or prepubescent female patients."

Alpha interferon: Marchand et al (2001) described the success of alpha interferon in treating a child with sight-threatening ocular complications, when azathioprine was ineffective, and when relapses occurred during prednisone tapering.[32]

Friedlander et al (2002) used ***fluticasone propionate 0.05% cream*** safely to treat pediatric skin conditions (in this case, atopic dermatitis) in children ranging in age from three months to six years. There were no apparent side effects when used for up to four weeks.[44]

Interested readers may also wish to refer to the following journal articles for **more information on treating children with rheumatic diseases** such as Behçet's:

Bloom BJ. ***New drug therapies for the pediatric rheumatic diseases***. Current Opinion in Rheumatology 2001; 13:410-414

Lepore L, Kiren V. ***Autologous bone marrow transplantation versus alternative drugs in pediatric rheumatic diseases***. Haematologica. 2000 Nov;85(11 Suppl):89-92

Wulffraat NM, Sanders LA, Kuis W. ***Autologous hemopoietic stem-cell transplantation for children with refractory autoimmune disease.*** Curr Rheumatol Rep. 2000 Aug;2(4):316-2

Klein-Gitelman MS, Pachman LM. ***Intravenous corticosteroids: adverse reactions are more variable than expected in children.*** J Rheumatol. 1998 Oct;25(10):1995-2002

Kurahara DK. ***Complementary medicine techniques to help reduce muscular pain in the pediatric rheumatic illnesses.*** Hawaii Med J 2001 Nov;60(11):289

Merkel SI, Gutstein HB, Malviya S. ***Use of transcutaneous electrical nerve stimulation [TENS] in a young child with pain from open perineal lesions.*** J Pain Symptom Manage 1999 Nov;18(5)376-81

Zangger EY, So A, Hofer M. P189: ***Use of alternative therapies in children with rheumatic diseases.*** Ann Rheum Dis - 60 (Supplement 2): 17ii [*It will be necessary to contact the author(s) for the actual article and additional references, as only the abstract is available through* Annals of the Rheumatic Diseases.*]*

A final comment on children, parents, and perception of pain:
It can be stressful and emotionally draining to raise a child with a chronic illness. With a heartfelt desire for their children to be

"normal," some parents may downplay or ignore their child's physical complaints. How often have adult BD patients heard exasperating comments such as: "snap out of it," "you'll feel better in the morning," and the infamous "there's nothing wrong with you...you look perfectly healthy"? Children with Behçet's are no different - both in the actual pain that they live with, and the frustration that they feel when their illness is not taken seriously.

Several studies have made it clear that parents consistently underestimate the amount of pain that their children are experiencing when they are ill.[45,46,47,48] Whether this is done out of fear, love, or a host of other possible emotions, the end result (according to Chambers et al) is the following: "Parents' underestimation of their child's pain may contribute to inadequate pain control."[45] That is because health care practitioners often rely on parents as "proxy respondents," giving information on behalf of their sick children.[48] Whenever possible, Epps et al [48] suggest that doctors "not rely on parents as sole informants for assessment of disability, well-being and pain." In other words, the children's complaints need to be heard, so that their lives can be made more comfortable.

A fitting example of this approach comes from Kim, the mother of an 8-year-old girl with BD, whose story was presented in the book ***You Are Not Alone: 15 People with Behçet's***:

> "If I had any advice to give to parents of other Behçet's kids, it would be this: try to live as normal a life as you can, and try not to dwell on the disease too much. And above all - if your kid is telling you something about how he or she is feeling, you need to hear it, because I think kids tell you right."[49]

One final topic concerns how chronically-ill children cope with pain, when they live with family members who are dealing with their own chronic pain conditions. A research study by Schanberg et al (2001) states that "parents who were more likely to seek treatment for their own pain, or more likely to report interference with recreational activities because of pain, had children with higher pain ratings and poorer health status as measured by the physician global assessment." This statement does not imply that parents and family members in pain should stay away from doctors in order to protect their children's health from going downhill. Instead, Schanberg suggests that pediatricians should ask parents about their current health, and levels of pain or disability, in order "to identify children at risk for developing maladaptive pain coping strategies, and higher levels of disease-related pain and disability."[50] Once these children are identified, then pediatricians can involve the parents in interventions that will help their children cope better with pain.

References:
1) Kone-Paut I, Bernard JL. Behçet's disease in children: a French nationwide survey. In "Behçet's Disease", c1993 Elsevier Science Publishers BV, Godeau and Wechsler (eds), pp385-389
2) Stark AC, Bhakta B, Chamberlain MA, Dear P, Taylor PV. Life-threatening

transient neonatal Behçet's disease. Brit J Rheum 1997;36:700-702
3) Lewis MA, Priestley BL. Transient neonatal Behçet's disease. Arch Dis Child 1986 Aug;61(8):805-6
4) Fam AG, Siminovitch KA, Carette S, From L. Neonatal Behçet's syndrome in an infant of a mother with the disease. Ann Rheum Dis, 1981;40(5):509-12
5) Thivolet J, Cambazard F, Genvo M-F. Grande aphtose neonatale de transmission maternelle. Ann Dermatol Venereol 1982;109:815-16
6) Fain O, Lachassine E et al. "Neonatal Behçet's disease" in Behçet's Disease, c1993 Elsevier Science Publishers BV, Godeau and Wechsler (eds), p399-402
7) El-Roeiy A, Shoenfeld Y. Autoimmunity and pregnancy. Am J Reprod Immunol Microbiol 1985 Sep;9(1):25-32
8) Chong SK, Wright VM, Nishigame T, Raafat F et al. Infantile colitis: a manifestation of intestinal Behçet's syndrome. J Pediatr Gastroenterol Nutr 1988 Jul-Aug;7(4):622-7
9) Kari JA, Shah V, Dillon MJ. Behçet's disease in UK children: clinical features and treatment including thalidomide. Rheumatology (Oxford) 2001 Aug;40(8):933-8
10) Kim DK, Chang SN, Bang D, Lee ES, Lee S. Clinical analysis of 40 cases of childhood-onset Behçet's disease. Pediatric Dermatology 11(2):95-101
11) Krause I, Uziel Y et al. Childhood Behçet's disease: clinical features and comparison with adult-onset disease. Rheumatology 1999;38:457-462
12) Eldem B, Onur C, Ozen S. Clinical features of pediatric Behçet's disease. J Pediatr Ophthalmol Strabismus 1998 May-Jun;35(3):159-161
13) Sarica R, Azizlerli G, Kose A, Disci R, Ovul C, Kural Z. Juvenile Behçet's disease among 1784 Turkish Behçet's patients. Int J Dermatol 1996 Feb;35(2):109-111
14) Yamazaki S, Koyano T. A case of pediatric Behçet's disease with intestinal involvement. J Dermatol 1999 , Mar;26(3):160-163
15) Pivetti-Pezzi P, Accorinti M, Abdulaziz MA, La Cava M, Torella M, Riso D. Behçet's disease in children. Ophthalmol 1995;39(3):309-14
16) Kone-Paut I. [Behçet's disease: pediatric features]. Article in French. Ann Med Interne (Paris) 1999 Nov;150(7):571-5
17) Kone-Paut I, Yurdakul S et al. Clinical features of Behçet's disease in children: an international collaborative study of 86 cases. J Pediatr 1998 Apr;132(4):721-5
18) Majeed HA. Differential diagnosis of fever of unknown origin in children. Curr Opin Rheumatol 2000 Sep;12(5):439-44
19) Krause I, Uziel Y, Guedj D et al. Mode of presentation and multisystem involvement in Behçet's disease: the influence of sex and age of disease onset. J Rheumatol 1998 Aug;25(8):1566-9
20) Fujikawa S, Suemitsu T. Behcet disease in children: a nationwide retrospective survey in Japan. Acta Paediatr Jpn 1997 Apr;39(2):285-9
21) Kone-Paut I, Chabrol B, Riss JM et al. Neurologic onset of Behçet's disease: a diagnostic enigma in childhood. J Child Neurol 1997 Jun;12(4):237-41
22) Vignola S, Nobili F, Picco P et al. Brain perfusion spect in juvenile neuro-behcet's disease. J Nucl Med 2001 Aug;42(8):1151-7
23) Hamuryudan V, Yurdakul S, Ozbakir F, Yazici H, Hekim H. Monozygotic twins concordant for Behçet's syndrome. Arthritis Rheum 1991 Aug;34(8):1071-2
24) Gul A, Inanc M, Ocal L, Aral O, Carin M, Konice M. HLA-B51 negative monozygotic twins discordant for Behçet's disease. Br J Rheumatol 1997 Aug; 36(8): 922-3
25) Villanueva JL, Gonzalez-Dominguez J, Gonzalez-Fernandez R, Prada JL, Pena J, Solana R. HLA antigen familial study in complete Behçet's syndrome affecting three sisters. Ann Rheum Dis 1993;52:155-157 (26) Aronsson A, Tegner E. Behçet's syndrome in two brothers. Acta Dermatovener (Stockholm) 63:73-74
27) Woodrow JC, Graham DR, Evans CC. Case report: Behçet's syndrome in HLA-identical siblings. Brit J Rheum 1990;29:225-227
28) Fenech FF, Soler NG. Behçet's syndrome with neurological manifestations in 0 sisters. Brit Med J 1968;2:473-474
29) Kone-Paut I, Gorchakoff A, Weschler B, Garnier JM, Touitou. Update on paediatric Behçet's disease in France. Ann Rheum Dis 59(9):746

30) Brik R, Shamali H, Bergman R. Successful thalidomide treatment of severe infantile Behcet disease. Ped Dermatology March/April 2002;18(2):143

31) Mitra S, Koul RL. Paediatric neuro-Behçet's disease presenting with optic nerve head swelling. Br J Ophthalmol 1999;83:1096

32) Marchand S, Tchaplyguine F, LeGallo B, Collet B, Lauras B, Berger C, Kone-Paut I. Uveitis, pediatric Behcet disease (BD) and alpha interferon. Ann Rheum Dis;60 (Supplement 2):17ii

33) Yasui K, Komiyama A, Takabayashi Y, Fujikawa S. Behçet's disease in children. J of Pediatrics Feb 1999;134(2):249-250

34) Hamza M. Juvenile Behçet's disease. In "Behçet's Disease", c1993 Elsevier Science Publishers BV, Godeau and Wechsler (eds), pp377-38

35) Shafaie N, Shahram F, Davatchi F, Akbarian M, Gharibdoost F, Nadji A. Behçet's disease in children. In "Behçet's Disease", c1993 Elsevier Science Publishers BV, Godeau and Wechsler (eds), pp381-383

36) Stringer DA, Cleghorn GJ, Durie PR, Daneman A, Hamilton JR. Behçet's syndrome involving the gastrointestinal tract-a diagnostic dilemma in childhood. Pediatr Radiol 1986;16(2):131-4

37) Yazici H, Tuzun Y, Pazarli H, Yurdakul S et al. Influence of age of onset and patient's sex on the prevalence and severity of manifestations of Behçet's syndrome. Ann Rheum Dis 1984;43(6):783

38) Bardak Y. Effects of age and sex on Behçet's disease. J of Rheum 1999;26(4):1008

39) Barash J, Sthoeger D, Ben-Zeev B. Behçet's disease in a child. Arthritis Rheumatism June 1991;34(6):791

40) Lang BA, Laxer RM, Thorner P, Greenberg M, Silverman ED. Pediatric onset of Behçet's syndrome with myositis: case report and literature review illustrating unusual features. Arthritis Rheumatism March 1990;33(3):418-425

41) Rakover Y, Adar H, Tal I, Lang Y, Kedar A. Behcet disease: long-term follow-up of three children and review of the literature. Pediatrics June 1989;83(6):986-92

42) Sarica R, Azizlerli G et al. Juvenile Behçet's disease among 1784 Turkish Behçet's patients. Int J Dermatol 1996;35:109-111

43) Yosipovitch G, Shohat B, Bshara J, Wysenbeek A, Weinberger A. Elevated serum interleukin 1 receptors and interleukin 1B in patients with Behçet's disease: correlations with disease activity and severity. Isr J Med Sci 1995;32:245-8

44) Friedlander SF et al. Fluticasone cream safe in children with atopic dermatitis. J Am Acad Dermatol 2002;46(3):387-393

45) Chamber CT, Reid GJ, Craig KD, McGrath PJ, Finley GA. Agreement between child and parent reports of pain. Clin J Pain 1998 Dec;14(4):336-42

46) Doherty E, Yanni G, Conroy RM, Bresnihan B. A comparison of child and parent ratings of disability and pain in juvenile chronic arthritis. J Rheumatol 1993 Spt;20(9):1563-6

47) Goodenough TB, Perrott DA, Champion GD, Thomas W. Painful pricks and prickle pains: is there a relation between children's ratings of venipuncture pain and parental assessments of usual reaction to other pains? Clin J Pain 2000 Jun;16(2):135-43

48) Epps HA, Utley M, Hurley M. P043. Level of agreement between parent and child ratings of disability, pain and well-being in juvenile idiopathic arthritis. Ann Rheum Dis - 60 (Supplement 2): 17ii

49) Zeis J. "Ann: Behçet's at 8." In "You Are Not Alone: 15 People with Behçet's." c1997, p11   (50) Schanberg LE, Anthony KK, Gil KM, Lefebvre JC, Kredich DW, Macharoni LM. Family pain history predicts child health status in children with chronic rheumatic disease. Pediatrics 2001 Sep;108(3):E47

51) Bessmertny O, Pham T. Thalidomide use in pediatric patients. Ann Pharmacother 2002 Mar;36(3):521-5

CHAPTER 6

Behçet's disease in families

Can Behçet's disease occur in families? The short answer is: Yes it can, although it's supposedly not common. This "uncommon" definition may seem incredible to any Behçet's patient whose child, parent or sibling is also suffering with BD symptoms. When Behçet's strikes more than one person in a family, it's typical to assume that other BD households must exist with the same problem. Indeed, many members of Behçet's support groups do report multiple cases in their own families, and consider familial situations to be common occurrences. However, in actuality, researchers have shown that the frequency of familial Behçet's varies greatly between countries. It is currently believed that genes are not the only required ingredient to create a case of Behçet's - one or more viral, bacterial or environmental "triggers" are also necessary to set off BD in someone who is genetically predisposed to developing it. These unknown triggers become especially important when one hears of genetically-unique family situations: for example, two sets of genetically-identical twin brothers in Turkey, where one brother in each set develops Behçet's while the other remains healthy.[9] There is obviously much more to the Behçet's question than a simple genetic answer.

Like some other aspects of Behçet's disease, the frequency of BD's appearance in families may be dependent upon where the patient lives. According to a literature review by Gul et al (2000), 2-3% of Japanese patients have immediate family members with BD, while 8-34% of BD patients in Turkey and the Middle East claim a Behçet's family history.[1] Gul's own study of 170 Turkish Behçet's patients found 31 (18%) with relatives displaying complete BD symptoms, while Hamza and Bardi (1993) surveyed 607 Tunisian patients and discovered only 23 (3.4%) with a positive family history.[2] In Korea (1988), Kim et al noted a 13% family occurrence rate.[8] Defining frequency rates as high or low may be in the eye of the beholder, however: Kone-Paut et al (1998) referred to a 15% rate of familial cases in their international study as "particularly frequent," and stated that "the high frequency of familial cases calls for further investigation of the immunogenetic factors that may favor early expression of the disease."[7]

A family with a history of Behçet's is more than an interesting curiosity: certain disease features may be unique to this situation. For example, Fresko et al reported *genetic anticipation* in 84% of the families in their 1998 research study. Genetic anticipation is "earlier disease onset or increase in disease severity, or both, in successive generations."[3] Fresko's study focused on parents with BD, who also had one or more children with the disease. Sixteen of the families had one parent and one child with Behçet's; one family had a BD parent with two Behçet's children; and an even more unfortunate family had a BD parent with three affected children. In a significant number of cases, Behçet's children experienced their first BD symptoms at a younger age than their parent(s) had [first symptoms of the children occurred at a mean age of 20.57 (7.47) years, vs. 33.29 (9.92) years for their parents.] In addition, children satisfied the diagnostic criteria for Behçet's [showed necessary symptoms for a diagnosis of "complete" Behçet's] at a younger age than their parents: a mean age of 21.2 (6.74) years for children vs. 36.4 (9.55) years for their parents. The first symptom to appear in the majority of parents and children was oral ulcers, and the disease did not seem to be more severe in one generation over the other.

In 1999, Kone-Paut et al made an interesting discovery: children who fulfilled the BD criteria before the age of 16 were more likely to have other family members with Behçet's, than were patients who fulfilled criteria after age 16. In addition, the "before 16" group met the BD criteria almost ten years earlier than the patients in the "over 16" group.[6] Treudler's study (1999) found that even pediatric BD patients who showed symptoms but didn't fulfill the criteria before age 16 had a greater probability of having another relative with BD, than patients who began the disease process as an adult.[15]

Familial Behçet's disease does not have to be limited to a single parent/child link. In 1976, Goolamali et al reported on a household where BD appeared through four successive generations.[4] Other studies have shown the variety of family relationships that can be involved in Behçet's. A combination of results from three reports (Gul 2000, Nishiyama 2000, Hamza 1993) provides the following information:[1,2,5]

Three treatment centers in Tunisia, Japan and Turkey reviewed the medical histories of their Behçet's patients, to find those who had family members with BD. 137 patients were chosen, and their relatives were examined. Follow-up determined that:

45	of the original patients' brothers also had Behçet's
27	sisters
14	cousins
22	mothers
11	fathers
5	"parents" (unspecified)
6	daughters
9	sons
13	uncles or aunts
2	nephews or nieces

Some other research findings on familial Behçet's are worth noting here:

A Japanese study (**Nishiyama et al, 2000**) divided 83 familial Behçet's patients into two groups: those with eye involvement and those without. They found that:[5]

1) 64% of patients with ocular lesions were positive for HLA-B51.

2) Only 14% of patients without ocular lesions were positive for HLA-B51

3) Among patients without ocular involvement, the familial relationship tended to be parent/child, especially mother/child, although the difference was not significant.

4) There is an increase in the number of female patients who have no ocular involvement, but who do have genital lesions.

5) The researchers suggest that clinical findings of BD in the Far East are beginning to resemble Western countries' results: fewer positive HLA-B51 tests, and more frequent genital ulcers.

A Turkish study (**Onal et al, 2001**) looked at five pairs of siblings who had eye involvement associated with Behçet's disease. There were three sister-brother pairs, one sister-sister pair, and one brother-brother pair.[10]

1) The sisters developed disease symptoms at an earlier age than their brothers; their prognosis was also worse than their brothers'.

2) Clinical symptoms in three of the five pairs of siblings progressed differently.

3) A recommendation was made that each child in this situation should receive individual treatment based on his/her own clinical status, without arbitrarily duplicating the brother's or sister's treatment, and without assuming that siblings will follow the same disease course.

In Scandinavia, **Fallingborg et al (1986)** found that three out of twelve members of one family had BD. Four of the twelve family members (including the three with BD) had recurrent mouth ulcers.[11]

1) All four family members with oral ulcers had the following HLA results: HLA-A2, B15, CW3, and DR4, although three of the four members had Behçet's and one didn't.

2) One additional relative had identical HLA results to those above, but had no evidence of Behçet's symptoms, including oral ulcers.

In Turkey, **Akpolat et al (1992)** looked at 137 Behçet's patients, and discovered that 27 of those BD cases were contained within twelve families. The researchers found: [12]

1) There was significantly less vascular involvement in the patients who had other family members with BD (7% of patients in the familial group had vascular involvement, vs. almost 29% of the non-familial patients).

2) HLA-B51(5) and HLA-A2 figured prominently in the test results of the familial groups: HLA-B51(5) was positive in

68% of the familial patients, and HLA-A2 was positive in 75% of those cases.

In Japan, **Nishiura et al (1996)** found a 3% occurrence of Behçet's in families: 18 patients out of 564 surveyed indicated that they had other family members with BD.[13]

1) More siblings had Behçet's than any other family relationship in the survey (for example, there were more brother-sister Behçet's pairs than mother-child).

2) 92% of the familial patients tested positive for HLA-B5, which was highly significant when compared with healthy Japanese subjects in the study, and with the non-familial BD cases.

3) Female patients in the Behçet's families tended to have a worse visual prognosis, with uveoretinitis appearing in both eyes

In Israel, **Arber et al (1991)** found that: [14]

1) HLA-B51 and HLA-B52 were associated with Behçet's disease in Israeli patients in their familial study (63% of patients were B51 positive; 21% were B52 positive).

2) Six out of 34 families in the study had more than one BD patient in the family. Of the family members who had Behçet's, 95% tested positive for B51 or B52.

3) Recurrent oral ulcers were common in families that contained at least one Behçet's patient.

All of the above studies dealt with standard family relationships: parent-child, sister-brother, brother-brother, etc. But what happens when Behçet's invades the unique world of identical twins? We might assume that identical (monozygotic) twins would share the same health problems, and in this first report, that appears to be the case: Hamuryudan et al (1991) wrote about identical twin brothers in Turkey who had been raised together in the same home. Both brothers developed Behçet's when they reached the age of 23, with almost identical symptoms: oral ulcerations, scrotal ulcers, ostiofolliculitis, and a positive pathergy reaction. The brothers were HLA-identical, with positive results for HLA-B5. Minor health differences involved erythema nodosum in one brother only, and a slight discrepancy in the levels of retinal involvement.[16]

In 1997, however, Gul et al wrote about two sets of identical twin brothers (also in Turkey) who had markedly different medical histories than the brothers described above. In the first case, twin boys were raised in the same home, but from the age of 14 worked at different jobs. One young man developed Behçet's symptoms at the age of 21: oral/genital ulcerations, posterior uveitis in both eyes, and a positive pathergy test. He eventually lost his vision due to frequent eye inflammation. At the time Gul's report was written, the twins had reached the age of 26; the other twin was still healthy, with only minor, occasional oral ulcerations. His pathergy tests have been consistently negative. Both brothers in this case are HLA-B51 negative.[9]

In his report, Gul also wrote of 45-year-old identical twin brothers who had grown up in the same house, sharing the same room until they were 25. One man received a Behçet's diagnosis on the basis of oral and genital ulcerations, folliculitis, arthritis, and a positive pathergy test. In contrast, his twin brother has been totally free of BD symptoms, with a negative pathergy test. Both brothers are HLA-B51 negative. These twins have an older brother, however, who is HLA-B51 positive and has had a full complement of Behçet's-related health problems since the age of 28. Gul et al concluded their report with a suggestion for larger research studies involving identical and fraternal twins, as well as further investigation into familial BD cases; they feel these cases will help to clarify the role of genetic (and other) factors that lead to the development of Behçet's in individuals and/or families.

Additional "sibling studies" of note include the following:

Villanueva et al (1993): Their report concerned a Spanish family whose three female offspring all have Behçet's disease, while their three male siblings are healthy. All six children are HLA-B51 positive, and the young women share identical HLA typing (A2, A11, B51, B44, Cw6, Cw5, DR4, DRw13, DRw53, DRw52, DQw7, and DQw6). The researchers suggest that the all-female BD contingent in this case may be due to some level of hormonal involvement, or to specific (and unknown) familial HLA associations.[17]

Aronsson and Tegner (1982): This report concerned two Scandinavian brothers who had lived apart in separate homes, with no contact, from the time that they were 1 and 7 years old. In 1978 (27 years later), both brothers developed Behçet's; one had enough health issues for a diagnosis of complete Behçet's, while the other was regarded as a case of incomplete Behçet's. Neither patient carries HLA-B51. The older brother has the following HLA typing: HLA-A2, B17, W21; the younger ("incomplete BD") sibling has A2, B12, W21.[18]

Woodrow, Graham and Evans (1990): The authors described two brothers who carried identical HLA markers, but whose disease progression affected different body systems. One brother's ocular involvement was so severe that his eye inflammations resulted in a permanent, and almost total, loss of vision. The other young man developed extreme pulmonary complications, and died as a result. Woodrow et al drew the following conclusion, which, once again, emphasized the importance of looking at multiple factors when researching Behçet's within families: "The fact that...the HLA haplotypes were identical [in this family], but the major manifestations were different, suggests that HLA-linked genes are only part of a complex pathogenesis [origin and development] of the different forms of Behçet's syndrome."[19]

References:
1) Gul A, Inanc M, Ocal L, Aral O, Konice M. Familial aggregation of Behçet's disease in Turkey. Ann Rheum Dis 2000;59:622-625 (August)
2) Hamza M, Bardi R. "Familial Behçet's disease" in Behçet's Disease, c1993

Elsevier Science Publishers BV, Wechsler and Godeau (Eds.), p 391-393

3) Fresko I, Soy M, Hamuryudan V, Yurdakul S, Yavuz S, Tumer Z, Yazici H. Genetic anticipation in Behçet's syndrome. Ann Rheum Dis 1998;57:45-48 (January)

4) Goolamali SK, Comaish JS, Hassanyeh F, Stephens A. Familial Behçet's syndrome. Br J Dermatol 1976 Dec;95(6):637-42

5) Nishiyama M, Nakae K, Umehara T. A study of familial occurrence of Behçet's disease with and without ocular lesions. Jpn J Ophthalmol 2001;45:313-316

6) Kone-Paut I, Geisler I, Wechsler B, Ozen S et al. Familial aggregation in Behçet's disease: high frequency in siblings and parents of pediatric probands. J Pediatr 1999 Jul;135(1):89-93

7) Kone-Paut I, Yurdakul S, Bahabri SA et al. Clinical features of Behçet's disease in children: an international collaborative study of 86 cases. J Pediatr 1998 Apr;132(4):721-5

8) Lee S, Bang D, Lee ES, Sohn S (Eds.). "Familial occurrence" in Behçet's Disease: A Guide to its Clinical Understanding. c2001 Springer-Verlag, p17

9) Gul A, Inanc M, Ocal L, Aral O, Carin M, Konice M. HLA-B51 negative monozygotic twins discordant for Behçet's disease. Brit J of Rheum 1997;36:922-23 (letter)

10) Onal S, Tugal-Tutkun I, Urgancioglu M, Gul A. Clinical course of ocular Behçet's disease in siblings. Ocul Immunol Inflamm 2001 Jun;9(2):111-24

11) Fallingborg J, Ambrosius Christensen L, Grunnet N. HLA antigens in a family with Behçet's syndrome. Acta Med Scand 1986;220(4):375-8

12) Akpolat T, Koc Y, Yeniay I et al. Familial Behçet's disease. Eur J Med Nov 1992;1(7):391-5

13) Hishiura K, Kotake S, Ichiishi A, Matsuda H. Familial occurrence of Behçet's disease. Jpn J Ophthalmol 1996;40(2):255-9

14) Arber N, Klein T, Meiner Z, Pras E, Weinberger A. Close association of HLA-B51 and B52 in Israeli patients with Behçet's syndrome. Ann Rheum Dis 1991 Jun;50(6):351-3

15) Treudler R, Orfanos CE, Zouboulis CC. Twenty-eight cases of juvenile-onset Adamantiades-Behcet disease in Germany. Dermatology 1999;199(1):15-19

16) Hamuryudan V, Yurdakul S, Ozbakir F, Yazici H. Monozygotic twins concordant for Behçet's syndrome. Arthritis Rheum 1991 Aug;34(8):1071-2

17) Villanueva JL, Gonzalez-Dominguez J, Gonzalez-Fernandez R, Prada JL, Solana R. HLA antigen familial study in complete Behçet's syndrome affecting three sisters. Ann Rheum Dis 1993;52:155-157

18) Aronsson A, Tegner E. Behçet's syndrome in two brothers. Acta Dermatovener (Stockholm) 1982;63:73-74

19) Woodrow JC, Graham DR, Evans CC. Case report: Behçet's syndrome in HLA-identical siblings. Br J of Rheum 1990;29:225-227

CHAPTER 7

Behçet's disease in the U.S.

Behçet's disease presents special challenges for patients living in the United States. Not only is there a shortage of doctors experienced in treating BD in this country, there is also a shortage of doctors willing to *consider* Behçet's as a possible diagnosis. Common discounting statements include "It's too rare," and "You can't have it because you're not from the Middle East." This attitude may be ill-advised if it prevents patients from receiving timely and appropriate care for their medical problems, before any permanent damage occurs. According to Calamia et al (2000):

> "While uncommon, we believe that Behçet's disease can be diagnosed in patients away from high prevalence areas. Centuries ago, the disorder was introduced to those along the silk route by travelers who carried with them the genes or agents responsible for the disease. In subsequent years, descendants of these early traders continued the exchange of these products along the roads of exploration, conquest and migration, which have been a part of the history of Europe and the New World. As a result, the disease can be considered worldwide in distribution."[1]

Few large-scale Behçet's research studies have taken place in the U.S. over the last several decades in comparison to countries where BD is prevalent. This discrepancy can be frustrating for American patients looking for "local" information and support. That is why it was especially heartening to find two papers providing an overview of Behçet's symptoms in U.S. patients: "Clinical Characteristics of United States Patients with Behçet's Disease" (Calamia et al, 2000) and Davis and Brissett's 1993 report on "Experiencing Behçet's Disease - A View from 245 Patients."

In the first report, **Calamia et al (2000)** studied the medical records of 164 Behçet's patients seen at the Mayo Clinic in Minnesota from 1985-1997.[1] The researchers were able to draw several conclusions from their review of 115 female and 49 male patients' charts:

1) U.S. patients had symptoms occurring at frequency rates similar to patients in other parts of the world.
2) In this U.S. study, Behçet's occurred more frequently in women than in men - in contrast to research results in Silk Route countries, where male patients are more common.

3) There is a possibility that, overall, U.S. patients experience a less severe form of Behçet's than patients who are found in countries where BD is common.

4) Despite previous reports of low positivity of pathergy tests in U.S. patients, the positive pathergy result in this study approached 30%. However, a limited number of subjects were tested for the phenomenon.

It is also interesting to note the differences in various symptom frequencies between U.S. women and men in Calamia's study:

Behcet's symptom frequencies in U.S. women and U.S.men[1]

Symptom	Women (115 total)		Men (49 total)		All Patients	
Oral ulcers	113	(98%)	48	(98%)	161	(98%)
Genital ulcers	101	(88%)	30	(61%)	131	(80%)
Uveitis	56	(49%)	27	(55%)	83	(51%)
Retinal vasc.	24	(21%)	8	(16%)	32	(20%)
Skin disease	71	(62%)	37	(76%)	108	(66%)
Pathergy	4 of 27 tested		4 of 27 tested		8:27 tested	
Synovitis	33	(29%)	11	(22%)	44	(27%)
Arthralgia	16	(14%)	5	(10%)	21	(13%)
Spondylitis	1	(1%)	1	(2%)	2	(1%)
Large vessel	17	(15%)	14	(29%)	31	(19%)
CNS	23	(20%)	14	(29%)	37	(23%)
GI	6	(5%)	7	(14%)	13	(8%)
Epididymitis	–		4	(8%)	4	(2%)

We can see that genital ulcers are more prevalent in the U.S. in women than in men, while men take the lead in symptoms that create the most serious illness: uveitis, large vessel disease, and CNS complications. In another report, Calamia and Davatchi (2000) looked at the sensitivity of the six different available Behçet's criteria, when used in diagnosing U.S. patients with BD. They found that the Iranian "*Classification Tree*" was statistically the most sensitive in identifying U.S. patients[2] - much more so, in fact, than the widely-accepted International Study Group criteria described on pages 10-11 of this book. An outline of the *Classification Tree* appears below:

The Iran Criteria *Classification Tree*[2] *[JZ adaptation]*

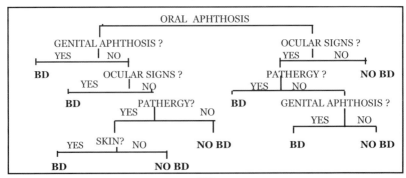

Moving on to **Davis and Brissett's 1993 report,**[3] the following statistics have been compiled from their research, in which 245 patients responded to a survey mailed to 616 members of the American Behçet's Disease Association. All of the responding patients were diagnosed between 1988-1992.

Respondents:
83%	female (5:1 female-to-male ratio)
93%	Caucasian
40%	diagnosed by rheumatologists
13%	diagnosed by dermatologists
13%	diagnosed by internists

There was an average of 7 years between patients' first BD-related symptoms, and their diagnosis. 21% of patients were diagnosed after 12 or more years of symptoms.

Disease Status:
32%	of respondents stated they had a "relatively mild case" of BD
37%	had a "moderate case" of Behçet's
31%	had a "relatively severe case" of Behçet's

Symptoms reported as most difficult to cope with: oral ulcers, pain, fatigue

Symptoms most reported as getting worse during flares: oral ulcers, arthritic pain, fatigue.

As general flare symptoms eased: 40% of respondents stated that oral ulcers decreased, but arthritic pain and fatigue stayed at moderate-to-severe levels.

According to Davis and Brissett: over time, "there is a tendency for flares to decrease in severity, frequency and duration, and for remissions to increase in frequency and duration, but symptom severity remains unchanged."

How life has changed for these patients since becoming ill:
(Listing is from "most affected" to "least affected" areas)
1) physical health is most affected
2) work activities
3) leisure activities
4) emotional health
5) relationships with family are least affected

73% of patients are less able to work because of weakness, fatigue, and/or pain levels. Only 14% of patients have been able to maintain their pre-illness activity levels.

Activities most frequently stopped due to illness:
team or competitive sports, and exercise

72% of respondents reported a change in physical appearance:
30% reported weight gain
19% reported "puffiness"
16% reported "facial change"

Disabilities:

50%   reported physical handicaps, with the majority reporting a decreased use of their limbs

20%   reported visual disabilities

12%   reported a handicapping level of fatigue and/or weakness

78%   of respondents use(d) assistance such as canes, handicapped parking permits, and/or vision aids

33%   of respondents applied for Social Security Disability payments. Of those who applied, 75% were approved, and 9% had cases pending.

Need for assistance from others:

44%   said that it took "minimal" effort to care for themselves

27%   reported a "moderate" level of effort for self-care

29%   reported a great deal of effort required for self-care

However, 75% of respondents stated that they **don't** require care from others on a regular basis

Most important sources of support:

1)   families
2)   relying on themselves
3)   spiritual beliefs
4)   American Behçet's Disease Association

Perceived causes for their disease:

33%   had no idea what had caused their disease

17%   considered the cause to be genetically-based

15%   felt that stress or lifestyle factors created their illness

13%   felt that their illness was caused by bacterial or viral agents

Most frequently prescribed medication (in 1993):

Prednisone, which patients also considered the most effective drug offerred

Perceived chances of disease being well-controlled in the future:
In spite of the wide range and severity of symptoms, almost half of these surveyed BD patients felt the chances were greater than 60% that their disease could be well-controlled in the future. According to the authors of the study, "Those respondents whose illness is most severe feel that the disease is least likely to be well controlled." In an important aside, the study's authors noted that "professionals were not viewed as supportive as one would hope."

References:

1) Calamia KT, Mazlumzadeh M, Balabanova M, Bagheri M, O'Duffy JD. Clinical characteristics of United States patients with Behçet's disease. Yonsei Medical Journal June 2000;Vol 41 Supplement, p9

2) Calamia KT, Davatchi F. Analysis of the sensitivity of diagnostic criteria in United States patients with Behçet's disease. Yonsei Medical Journal June 2000;Vol 41 Supplement, p9

3) Davis GL, Brissett D. Experiencing Behçet's disease: a view from 245 patients. In "Behçet's Disease," c1993 Elsevier Science Publishers, Wechsler and Godeau (Eds.), p211-214

CHAPTER 8

Ocular disease, cataracts, and treatment

The following articles have been reprinted with the permission of C. Stephen Foster, M.D., F.A.C.S., Director of the Ocular Immunology and Uveitis Service of the Massachusetts Eye and Ear Infirmary in Boston. Dr. Foster is on the Medical Advisory Board of the American Behçet's Disease Association, and has extensive experience treating the eye inflammations and disorders associated with Behçet's. His most recent book, *Diagnosis and Treatment of Uveitis* (c2002 WB Saunders Company, Eds: Foster and Vitale) is an exhaustively-detailed and meaty 900-page textbook, with a full chapter on the treatment of Adamantiades-Behcet disease.

 The articles in this chapter appear as part of MEEI's comprehensive Ocular Immunology web site, located at **www.uveitis.org**. The Ocular Immunology Service may be contacted through their web site, or by the following means: **Telephone**: (617) 573-5549 **Fax**: (617) 573-3181 **Postal Address**: Ocular Immunology Service, Massachusetts Eye & Ear Infirmary, 243 Charles Street, Boston, MA 02114 USA.

The information provided here is designed to support, and not replace, the relationship that exists between a patient and his/her existing physician.

Systemic Treatment of Ocular Disease
C. Stephen Foster, M.D.

Most eye diseases which are treatable are treated with eye drops. In fact, the number of instances in which patients attending a general ophthalmologist's office might be prescribed a systemic medication (i.e., one which is taken, for example, by mouth) is vanishingly small. Perhaps because of this and other factors, most ophthalmologists eventually consider treating patients with an eye problem only rarely with systemic medication. And while this is usually perfectly appropriate, in some instances, such as in the care of patients with uveitis, we believe that to neglect strong consideration of systemic therapy for the condition is to ensure that no progress will be made in reducing the prevalence of blindness secondary to the disease. Indeed, the evidence on the subject of uveitis is clear: the prevalence of blindness caused by this disease has not been reduced in the past thirty years; it remains the number three cause of preventable blindness in the United States.

Eye drops (steroids) remain the mainstay and cornerstone of reatment of patients with uveitis. But some patients with uveitis continue to have episodes of active inflammation each time the topical steroid drops are reduced and discontinued. All ophthalmologists realize that they cannot keep their patient with uveitis on topical steroids indefinitely; cataract is a guaranteed side effect from the chronic use of steroid eye drops; glaucoma is a significant possibility from such use; and increased susceptibility to eye infections, including those from herpes simplex virus, is also a risk. The all-too-frequent scenario, therefore, is: Treatment of the uveitis with steroid drops, resolution of the uveitis, tapering and discontinuation of the steroid drops, recurrence of the uveitis, reinstitution of steroid eye drop therapy, etc.

We believe that there is a better way, and, in fact, the "outcomes" study data show that this is so. Our philosophy, on the Immunology and Uveitis Service at the Massachusetts Eye and Ear Infirmary over the past two decades has been to not tolerate even low-grade chronic uveitis, but also not to tolerate endless amounts of steroid use. We achieve this goal through a "stepladder" approach in aggressiveness of therapy. The next "step" on this stepladder, after topical steroids, is oral nonsteroidal anti-inflammatory drug therapy. This class of drug, nonsteroidal anti-inflammatory drugs, is typified by aspirin, ibuprofen, naproxen, etc. Unless a patient has a contraindication to the use of such medications chronically by mouth (for example, history of peptic ulcer disease), we place the patient on prescription-strength nonsteroidal anti-inflammatory drugs, and then attempt to taper the topical steroid drops, expecting the oral nonsteroidal medication to keep the uveitis from recurring. This strategy, in our hands, is effective in approximately 70% of selected patients. In those 30% who do not respond to this strategy, we then advance to systemic immunosuppressive/immuno-modulatory therapy, sometimes referred to as "chemotherapy." I place this word in quotation marks simply because it is not the kind of chemotherapy that most patients think of when they hear that word, i.e., cancer-type therapy. Rather, it is the type of chemotherapy typically used by rheumatologists in their care of patients with severe rheumatoid arthritis, and by dermatologists in their care of patients with severe psoriasis, or in their care of patients with certain blistering dermatitis diseases.

This is the area in systemic drug therapy for ocular disease in which the vast majority of ophthalmologists are uncomfortable, primarily out of ignorance (and I do not mean that in a pejorative way, but rather in a factual way.) Ophthalmologists are not used to using these medications, and carry with them the "baggage" learned in Medical School about the risks of immunosuppressive chemotherapy drugs, typically as they are used in solid organ transplant patients and in patients with malignant disease. And those risks are simply not the same as the risks associated with the low-dose, single-agent immuno-suppressive chemotherapeutic programs that rheumatologists, derma-tologists, and ocular immunologists use in their care of patients with non-malignant inflammatory disease. The potential for drug-induced "mischief" exists; but, used correctly, the likelihood of a significant drug-induced problem is quite small. The drugs, of course, must be managed by an individual who is, by virtue of training and experience, an expert in their use, in a patient who is responsible, keeps his or her appointments, etc.

We believe that unless or until increasing numbers of ophthalmologists embrace the idea of systemic therapy for certain blinding ocular diseases, the prevalence of blindness from such diseases will go unchanged, as it has over the past 30 years.

Cataract Surgery and Uveitis
C. Stephen Foster, M.D.

Cataract develops in patients with uveitis because of the uveitis itself, and also because of the steroids which are the cornerstone of treating uveitis. Cataract developing in an eye with a history of chronic or recurrent uveitis has historically been called cataracta complicata, and, indeed, the uveitic cataract is a complicated cataract. It is complicated both from the standpoint of technical aspects of the surgery itself (limited access secondary to posterior synechiae, pupillary membrane, and pupillary sphincter sclerosis, iris delicacy and vascular abnormalities, and pre-existing glaucoma), and also because of the high likelihood of an exuberant postoperative inflammatory response which can ruin the desired surgical outcome. But the increasing availability of more delicate microsurgical techniques, through the use of pupil expanders, visco elastic material, small incision phacoemulsification techniques, etc. has dramatically reduced the misadventures that used to be so common. Yet, despite these advances surgeons are frequently still disappointed with the visual outcome of cataract surgery in the patient with a history of uveitis. This typically occurs as a result of two things: damage done to the macula or optic nerve long before the time for cataract surgery has arrived (through the consequences of recurrent or chronic, even "low grade" inflammation); and significant ongoing chronic or recurrent inflammation which sabotages an initially good visual result from cataract surgery.

Both these problems are avoidable, but avoidance of structural damage to areas of the eye critical for good vision requires a philosophy, on the ophthalmologists' part, of total intolerance to chronic or recurrent inflammation, achieving the goal of complete freedom of inflammation through a stepladder algorithm approach in aggressiveness of therapy. Indeed, prevention of cataract development in the first place often derives from such a philosophy. And postoperative inflammatory damage which sabotages an initially good visual outcome occurs, generally, if the patient is prepared ahead of surgery with treatment techniques that prevent exuberant inflammation postoperatively, and prevent a recurrence of inflammation or a continued low grade chronic inflammation longitudinally following surgery.

The exact details of surgical technique, above and beyond the routine required for adequate access to the lens and control of inflammation is very much patient and disease-specific. For example, many (indeed, perhaps even most) patients with a history of uveitis can have, as part of the surgical plan, implantation of a posterior chamber intraocular lens implant; exceptions to this generalization exist, for example, in most patients with uveitis on the basis of juvenile rheumatoid arthritis (JRA), and in patients for whom recurrent inflammation episodically through time is unpredictable and generally not preventable (i.e., patients with sarcoidosis, or even with patients with a history of multiple recurrences of toxoplasma retino-choroiditis.) Also, the exact details of which glaucoma procedure to perform, in the patient who needs glaucoma surgery in conjunction with cataract surgery, is also somewhat disease-specific and patient-dependent. And, finally the issue of simultaneous pars plana vitrectomy is very much disease-dependent. We believe, for example, that most patients with JRA-associated iridocyclitis and patients with pars planitis or uveitis that has been characterized by great "vitritis" or multiple recurrences affecting the posterior segment very much benefit from primary pars plana vitrectomy at the time of the cataract surgery. For further reading on this subject may I suggest the following references:

1) Foster CS, Barrett F: Cataract Development and Cataract Surgery in Patients with Juvenile Rheumatoid Arthritis-associated Iridocyclitis. Ophthalmology 1993; 100:809-817.
2) Foster CS, Fong LP, Singh G: Cataract Surgery and Intraocular Lens Implantation in Patients with Uveitis. Ophthalmology 1989; 96:281-288.
3) Foster RE, Lauder CY, Meisler DM, et al: Extracapsular cataract extraction with posterior chamber intraocular lens implantation in uveitis patients. Ophthalmology 1992; 99:1234-1241.
4) Gee SS, Tabbara KF: Extracapsular cataract extraction in Fuchs' heterochromic iridocyclitis. Am J Ophthalmol 1989; 108:310-314.
5) Kaufman AH, Foster CS: Cataract extraction in pars planitis patients. Ophthalmology 1993; 100:1210-1217.
6) Seamone CD, Deschenes J, Jackson WB: Cataract extraction in uveitis: comparison of aphakia and posterior chamber lens implantation. Can J Ophthalmol 1992; 273:1231-124.

*[JZ: In a recent study by Kadayifcilar, Gedik, Eldem and Irkec (**Cataract surgery in patients with Behçet's disease**. J Cataract Refract Surg 2002 Feb;28(2):316-20) the authors state the following: "In patients with Behçet's disease, inflammation after extracapsular surgery was mild when surgery was performed after at least 3 months of no inflammatory signs." There was no difference in amount of postoperative inflammation according to the type of surgery performed: ECCE, ECCE with IOL implantation, or phacoemulsification with IOL implantation.]*

Cataract Surgery and Recovery

The [cataract] surgery itself is generally done on an outpatient basis, and typically takes anywhere from 15 to 30 minutes to perform. A small incision is made for removal of the cataract and, generally, an artificial lens (lens implant) is placed in the eye after the cataract has been removed. The eye is patched, and the patient is typically asked to return for re-evaluation the following day to make certain that everything is perfect, and to begin with the post-operative medications (drops) that are typically prescribed following cataract surgery. The patient may see extremely well the moment the patch is removed on the day after surgery. In some instances, it may take several weeks for the patient to enjoy the full benefits of improved vision following the surgery.

Restrictions in physical activity following surgery are generally minimal, and are limited to restrictions on activities which could dramatically raise the pressure in the eye (bending at the waist to lift something heavy), activities that could result in exertion of pressure on the outside of the eye (sleeping with the eye pressed against the hand or pillow), and extremely vigorous jarring activity (for example jogging). Medications are generally tapered and discontinued within a relatively short period after surgery, and glasses for seeing the sharpest that the eye can possibly see, both at distance and at near, are then prescribed. Only one eye is generally operated upon at a time. Assuming that things go extremely well with the surgery, the other eye may appropriately have surgery relatively soon after the first eye has been successfully rehabilitated.

Surgical Cases Requiring IOL Explantation [Removal]

Most uveitis experts have agreed over the past decade that an in-the-bag posterior chamber IOL (PC-IOL) can be well tolerated in patients with a history of uveitis provided the uveitis has been perfectly quiet for a sustained period prior to surgery and provided that the uveitis remains inactive after surgery. However, complications associated with the use of lens implants continue to cause serious problems, leading in some instances to the need for removal of the IOL. We reviewed the clinical records of 1463 patients with uveitis treated on the Immunology Service of the Massachusetts Eye and Ear Infirmary during a period of 20 years. All clinical evaluations were performed by the same physician (Dr. Foster). We identified those patients who had had cataract surgery with IOL implantation (at this hospital or elsewhere) and those who had subsequently had the IOL removed.

Nineteen patients had IOL explantation [removal] over the 20-year period. The mean age of the patients was 42 years, with a range of 5 to 69 years. Fourteen patients were female and five were male. Twelve were white, six were black, and one was Asian. The uveitis was non-granulomatous in eight patients and granulomatous in eleven. The most common location was panuveitis (12 patients); six patients had intermediate uveitis and one anterior uveitis. The most common diagnoses were sarcoidosis, juvenile rheumatoid arthritis, and pars planitis. The average duration of the uveitis was 146 months (range 44 to 312 months). The average follow-up time was 60 months (range 5 to 147 months). Seven eyes (37%) improved two or more lines of Snellen acuity after IOL explantation. Five eyes had no improvement in vision, but the progressive degradation of vision pre-operatively was halted. The vision in seven eyes continued to deteriorate after IOL explantation. Only nine patients, of these nineteen, had control of the inflammation prior to cataract surgery for at least 2 1/2 months. Ten did not have any supplemental pre-operative preparation with any topical or systemic anti-inflammatory medication before surgery. The average interval from implantation to IOL removal was 28 months (range 2 to 91 months). The most frequent reasons for IOL removal were uncontrolled inflammation, and membrane formation with progressive hypotony.

Five of the nineteen patients described in this report were our patients from the Uveitis Service of the Massachusetts Eye and Ear Infirmary. We thought we were easily able to discriminate between those patients who could safely and those who could not safely have a lens implant placed at the time of removal of uveitic cataract. Clearly this was not so. The results of this study show, we believe, that patients with the inflammation affecting the intermediate region of the eye, and especially those with systemic disease which is unlikely to be cured or "burn out" soon, are at an especially high risk for IOL intolerance, with membrane formation, membrane contraction, progressive hypotony, and/or uncontrolled inflammation. Removal of an IOL in a patient with IOL intolerance after uveitic cataract surgery should probably be done sooner rather than later. Young JRA patients in particular probably should not even be considered for lens implantation associated with the removal of their cataract.

Pediatric Uveitis
C. Stephen Foster, M.D.

Uveitis is the third leading cause of blindness in America, and 5% to 10% of the cases occur in children under the age of 16. But uveitis in children blinds a larger percentage of those affected than in adults, since 40% of the cases occurring in children are posterior uveitis, compared to the 20% of posterior uveitic cases in the adult uveitis population.

There are, at any one time, approximately 115,000 cases of pediatric uveitis in the United States, with 2,250 new cases occurring each year. Spread across the entire U.S. population, therefore, and across all offices of ophthalmic practitioners, the likelihood that any one individual practitioner will care for a patient with pediatric uveitis is relatively small, and the likelihood that any single individual will have significant experience in caring for large numbers of cases over a long period of time is vanishingly small. This accounts, we believe, at least in part for the sub-optimal care that many of our children with uveitis appear to be receiving, even in these "modern" times. The stakes are incredibly high: for the child, for the parents who will be faced with (usually) many years of dealing with this health problem in their child, and for society at large because of the lifetime of dependence which occurs in those who eventually reap substantial visual handicap as the result of sub-optimal treatment.

We believe that current epidemiologic data emphasize two critically important goals for all of us in Ophthalmology, acting together, in an effort to change the current prevalence of blindness caused by pediatric uveitis:

> Repeatedly emphasizing to parents and other medical colleagues, especially pediatricians and school personnel, the critical importance of routine (annual) vision screening for all children.

> The critical importance of beating back the frontiers of general ignorance and mind sets, eliminating the all-too-common pronouncement by physicians to parents of a child with pediatric uveitis that:
> 1) "He'll/she'll outgrow it."
> 2) "The drops will get him (her) through it."
> 3) "It's just the eye; systemic therapy is not warranted."

Statements (1) and (2) are true, but too often pull the doctor, patient, and family into the seduction of nearly endless amounts of topical steroid therapy. It is generally true that the child will in fact "outgrow" the uveitis, i.e., that the uveitis will no longer be a problem eventually. The pity is, however, that so often by the time the child "outgrows it," permanent structural damage to retina, optic nerve, or aqueous outflow pathways has already occurred, and the blinding consequences are now permanent. It is also true that for any individual episode of uveitis, the steroid drops usually will get the patient through it. But the fact is that so many children with pediatric uveitis have recurrent episodes of uveitis such that the cumulative damage caused by each episode of uveitis and the steroid therapy for each episode eventually produces vision-robbing damage. And item (3) is simply the result of the common myopic viewpoint of ophthalmologists: that it is just an eye problem, and therefore should simply be treated with eye medications. Nothing could be further from the truth! And unless and until large numbers of ophthalmologists reframe this socially and epidemiologically important matter, the prevalence of blindness secondary to pediatric uveitis is not going to change.

The differential diagnosis of pediatric uveitis is relatively vast, and therefore the detective work required to properly pursue the underlying diagnosis is complex. We believe that aggressive efforts should be made to uncover the underlying cause of uveitis in any child. If the review of systems is negative and the patient has non-recurrent anterior granulomatous uveitis, we would not do laboratory studies. However, if review of systems is positive, we would "follow the review of systems."

For recurrent anterior non-granulomatous uveitis: we would obtain a complete blood count and urine analysis, ANA testing, HLA-B27 testing, and would "follow the review of systems."

The diagnostic stepladder in a pediatric patient with anterior granulomatous uveitis, recurrent or not, would include a CBC with urine analysis, and FTA-ABS testing, Lyme disease antibody and western block, PPD analysis, chest X-ray, ANA, and angiotensin converting enzyme determination. Chest CT, and Gallium scanning would be pursued if diagnosis of sarcoidosis was strongly suspected, and, of course as usual, we would "follow the review of systems positives." In a patient with intermediate uveitis, all would deserve laboratory evaluation, including CBC, urine analysis, chest X-ray, FTA-ABS, ACE, PPD, Lyme, and ANA titers.

Any patients with posterior uveitis would deserve an extensive vasculitis work-up, if vasculitis were present, and a search for "the usual suspects" with an eye to an infectious etiology, such as that producing a granuloma in the choroid in a patient with toxocariasis or toxoplasmosis. An audiogram or lumbar puncture would be done if positive [results] on the review of systems were found, such as tinnitus and/or meningeal signs or symptoms. Finally, a diagnostic vitrectomy would be added to the step ladder in a patient with posterior uveitis if all non-invasive studies were unrevealing and the case was difficult to treat successfully.

On the matter of **treatment**, here too we believe strongly in the stepladder approach, always beginning with steroids, in any route required to achieve the desired goal, i.e., abolition of all active inflammation. Topical steroids would be followed by an examination under anesthesia with regional steroid injection therapy in a patient with granulomatous or non-granulomatous anterior uveitis. Systemic steroids would be employed in the event that this approach did not achieve the goal of abolition of all active cells. We are extremely reluctant to get involved with long-term daily systemic steroid use in a youngster, because of the obvious growth-retarding properties of such therapy. But long-term oral non-steroid anti-inflammatory drug therapy, managed by a pediatrician, can be extremely successful, in our experience, in approximately 70% of children with recurrent non-granulomatous anterior uveitis. If this strategy is not successful, then consideration of once-weekly, low-dose, Methotrexate or daily Cyclosporine would be the next considerations.

In granulomatous disease topical steroids often are not sufficient, and systemic therapy, particularly with oral non-steroidal inflammatory drugs, may be utilized sooner rather than later. With intermediate uveitis [pars planitis], topical steroids are not effective in penetrating to the level of inflammatory focus. Regional steroid injections or systemic steroids are employed to treat that area, sometimes with adjunctive topical steroids for anterior chamber "spill-over" reaction. Retinal cyropexy can be effective in selected cases of recurrent pars planitis, as can therapeutic pars plana vitrectomy. Systemic immunomodulatory therapy, as usual, represents the final step in the step-ladder approach in the aggressiveness of care. Patients with posterior uveitis of course do not respond to topical therapy, and therefore require systemic steroids and/or immunomodulators right from the very beginning.

We hope that this [information] will provide some help to those ophthalmologists who have also concluded that the usual approach to pediatric uveitis, i.e., steroid drops, is not always sufficient, but who are hesitant to take the initiative to commit the patient to more aggressive treatment.

Retinal Vasculitis: Its Significance
C. Stephen Foster, M.D.

Unlike uveitis in the absence of retinal vasculitis, a situation in which approximately 30% of cases may turn out to be idiopathic [no known cause], uveitis associated with retinal vasculitis is almost never idiopathic. Further, the disease causing the ocular inflammation is nearly invariably a systemic one. The systemic disease is often occult [hidden], defying even the best internist's efforts at uncovering the "cause" of the patient's uveitis and retinal vasculitis. But through time, extraocular manifestations of the patient's systemic disease eventually emerge, making quite clear the nature of the underlying systemic disease. Polyarteritis nodosa, Wegener's ganulomatosis, systemic lupus erythematosus, sarcoidosis, multiple sclerosis, Behcet's disease, and syphilis are but a few of the diseases that can behave in this way.

Furthermore, the significance of the de novo appearance of retinal vasculitis in the patient with a well-established systemic disease is also profound. For example, a patient with well-characterized **Behcet's disease** with oral and genital ulcers, arthritis, and erythema nodosum may be well-controlled and highly functional on twice daily colchicine, an oral non-steroidal anti-inflammatory agent, and low-dose prednisone. The appearance of retinal vasculitis carries with it profound implications for such a patient. The aforementioned therapeutic "recipe" will no longer be sufficient for this patient. The appearance of the retinal vasculitis is a signal the underlying character of the patient's Behcet's disease has now changed, and unless the vigor of treatment is increased, not only is the patient likely to be bilaterally blind within four years, but the patient has approximately a 30% chance of developing vasculitis of the brain as well. Similar phenomena exist with respect to patients with systemic lupus erythematosus, rheumatoid arthritis, relapsing polychondritis, Wegener's granulomatosis, and polyarteritis nodosa.

The significance of the presence of retinal vasculitis, therefore is enormous, both from the standpoint of the likelihood of eventually discovering an underlying systemic disease causing the retinal vasculitis and also from the standpoint of the retinal vasculitis being a "barometer" of sub-clinical vasculitic lesions that may be lethal if the patient is not more vigorously treated.

Dry Eye
C. Stephen Foster, M.D.

Keratoconjunctivitis sicca syndrome (KCS or dry eye) is a problem of major epidemiologic importance. It affects literally millions of people around the globe, with women dramatically over-represented, particularly those women who have entered menopause. The problem may accompany dry mouth, and may be found in association with a systemic disease such as rheumatoid arthritis or systemic lupus erythematosus. It is, in many instances, far more than a simple "nuisance" problem. It has the potential for serious ocular consequences, beginning with the formation of dry spots on the cornea, progressing to epithelial defects or "abrasions" which resist healing, and then in some instances eventuating to ulceration of the cornea, sometimes even with frank perforation.

The mainstay of treatment for dry eye syndrome through the years has been replacement of fluid through the use of artificial tears. And while this is an important approach to the treatment of dry eye, it is by no means the only (or perhaps even the most important) approach. Conservation measures are also extremely important: the use of punctum plugs to reduce the loss of fluid from the eye through the nasolacrimal duct into the lacrimal sac and then down the throat; the use of side shield panels on spectacles to reduce the amount of air flow across the cornea and hence reduce evaporation; and the use of humidification techniques at home, again, in an effort to reduce the rate of loss of fluid from the surface of the eyes through evaporation. Additionally, we strongly believe that increasing the flow of oil from the oil ducts in the eyelids that supply a thin film of oil to the preocular tear film is extremely useful and important in the care of patients with KCS. Almost every patient whom I see with dry eye has a significant contribution from the oil component of the tear film being deficient. The use of warm compresses twice daily with gentle lid massage to dilate the oil ductules in the lids, further liquefy the oil, which sometimes "sets up" like toothpaste inside the oil ducts, promotes continual flow of oil to the tear film, producing a much more stable tear film, and a tear film which is much more efficient at keeping the surface of the eye lubricated, retarding evaporation of the liquid from the surface of the eye, and promoting more uniform spreading of the tear film across the entire extent of the ocular surface. Finally, the use of specially constructed scleral lenses *[JZ: see article on **Contact Lenses**, at www.uveitis.org]* can additionally be helpful in retaining a layer of liquid against the cornea in patients who have profound lack of adequate tears.

Behçet's Disease: An Overview

Esen Karamursel Akpek, M.D.
Immunology Service, Massachusetts Eye & Ear Infirmary

Systemic Findings

Recurrent **aphthous stomatitis** is a "sine qua non" of BD, and is usually the first systemic manifestation. They are typically round, sharply defined, painful and usually localized on the lips, gingiva, buccal mucosa, tongue and less commonly on the palate, tonsils and pharynx. They usually heal within 7 to 10 days. [13]

    Genital ulcers in male patients may appear on the scrotum and penis; in female patients lesions can develop on the vulva or vagina. They tend to be deeply located and often scar. An examination of the genital region can therefore be diagnostically useful in a suspected BD patient. [13] **Other skin lesions** typical of BD include erythema nodosum on the anterior surface of the legs, acneiform lesions or pseudofolliculitis on the backs and faces of the patients, and migratory thrombophlebitis.[14] Another dermatologic feature of BD is the positive **pathergy test**. In this test a sterile skin prick is performed with a sterile needle. The presence of marked redness and swelling, or a pustular lesion 24 to 48 hours later is interpreted as a positive result. Among American and Western Europian patients the positivity rate is extremely low. Among Turks it is positive in 79% of patients with vascular system disease and 56% in patients without vascular disease, indicating a significant association of positive pathergy tests with vascular involvement.[15]

    At least half of the patients are affected by non-migratory, non-destructive **arthritis**. It usually reflects the level of systemic disease activity and is occasionally linked to ocular lesions. **Vaso-occlusive inflammatory changes** with aneurysm or thrombus formation can affect vessels of all sizes and can be life threatening. **CNS manifestations** of BD can be global or focal and can cause sensory, motor, or neuropsychiatric symptoms. Meningoencephalitis is the most common form of CNS involvement.

Ocular Findings

Ophthalmic involvement can be the presenting symptom of BD. A review of a Japanese patient population suggests that ocular involvement is more common in males (83 to 95%) than in females (67 to 73%), and that the incidence of ocular symptoms as the initial manifestation of BD is higher in male (24.5%) than in female (8.6%) patients .[16] Also CNS involvement with its potentially fatal sequela correlates with ocular involvement. Although unilateral ocular manifestations do occur, ocular involvement is usually bilateral, often asymmetric.

    The classic finding in ocular BD is recurrent, sterile **hypopyon** [pus in the anterior chamber] described by Behçet, and it is a dramatic finding that is easily detected by non-ophthalmic physicians. However it only occurs in 1/3 of cases .[16] The patient complains of periorbital pain, redness, photophobia, and blurred vision. Slit-lamp biomicroscopy shows conjunctival and ciliary injection, with aqueous flare and cells. Fine keratic precipitates are present on the corneal endothelium. The attack lasts 2 to 3 weeks, then subsides. But recurrences are the rule, with subsequent iris atrophy and posterior synechia formation. Rare anterior segment findings include corneal immune ring opacity, conjunctival ulcers, episcleritis and scleritis. [17, 18]

The classic fundus finding is the necrotizing, obliterative **retinal vasculitis** affecting both arteries and veins in the posterior pole.[7] Vascular sheathing with perivascular exudates, arteriolar attenuation, venous dilatation and tortuosity, and branch and central retinal vein occlusion are common posterior pole findings. Vitritis is always present during the acute phase. Fluorescein angiography is useful in determining the extent of retinal and disc vasculitis. Typically there is leakage of dye from the small venules. In a recent Turkish study fundus angiographic abnormalities were found in 93% of cases with BD. In the same study abnormal leakage of dye from peripheral retinal capillaries and venules was found in 6% of patients who had no visual complaints as well as no abnormal findings on fundus exam.[19]

Cataract formation is the most common anterior segment complication after recurrent inflammation, occurring in up to 36% of cases.[20] It was reported that the post-operative visual acuity was found to be significantly lower in eyes with BD than in those with idiopathic uveitis because of the severe posterior segment complications, mainly optic atrophy. [21] Posterior synechiae, iris atrophy, and peripheral anterior synechia may develop during the course of repeated ocular inflammatory attacks. Peripheral anterior synechia or iris bombé from pupillary seclusion may cause secondary glaucoma. Retinal atrophy with optic atrophy is the end result of repeated episodes of posterior segment inflammation.

[JZ: Interested readers should also see the following article by Evereklioglu and Er: **Increased corneal thickness in active Behçet's disease.** *Eur J Ophthalmol 2002 Jan-Feb;12(1):24-9.]*

Pathology and Pathogenesis
The ocular histopathologic changes are basically identical to those occurring in other organs , that is necrotizing, leukocytoclastic obliterative vasculitis which is probably immune complex mediated and affects both arteries and veins of all sizes. During acute inflammation, the ciliary body and choroid show diffuse infiltration with neutrophils. During remission, infiltration with lymphocytes and plasma cells is seen. In late, chronic stages, there is proliferation of collagen fibers, sometimes with formation of a cyclitic membrane thickening of the choroid and sometimes hypotony and phthisis bulbi.

Tissue damage in BD is caused by aberrant HLA-DR expression, immune complex deposition within the blood vessel wall and activation of complement system and vasculitis. Abnormalities of neutrophil functions, such as enhanced migration and generation of free radicals, and elevated levels of circulating activated T lymphocytes have been reported.[22, 23] Sakane and associates reported a defect in the T-lymphocyte-mediated suppressor system and alterations in the CD4/CD8 ratio of circulating cells of patients with BD, which can be explained by an increase in the CD8 fraction of T-lymphocytes.[24] IL-8 levels were found to be higher in patients with active BD in a recent study, and since IL-8 has a potent effect on neutrophils, they concluded that this cytokine most likely participates in the inflammatory response of this disease.[25]

Laboratory Investigations

There are no laboratory findings specific for BD, and therefore careful assessment of a patient's clinical findings and history are critical for diagnosis. Patients may have high ESR, CRP or increased numbers of peripheral leukocytes during the active stages of the disease. The presence of autoantibodies or extremely high values of immunoglobulin are not compatible with a diagnosis of BD; instead they suggest collagen vascular disease.

The pathergy test can be useful, and in fact it is one of the criteria suggested by the ISG [International Study Group for Behçet's Disease].

Differential Diagnosis

In patients with the incomplete form of BD or with an atypical presentation it is important to consider other forms of uveitis in the differential diagnosis.

In systemic lupus erythematosus, the retinal vasculitis is in the form of obliterative arteriolitis. The retinal vasculitis of BD tends to be hemorrhagic rather than obliterative and involves arteries and veins. The appearance of the retina in BD can be similar to the appearance of viral retinitis; in both processes there is patchy retinal infarction. Retinal infiltrates in BD do not progress to coalesce, and hemorrhagic vascular occlusion and the presence of branch retinal vein occlusion are not typical of viral retinitis. The hypopyon associated with HLA-B27-associated uveitis is less mobile than BD-associated hypopyon because of the increased fibrinous reaction and it is usually unilateral. Systemic vasculitic diseases should also be considered in the differential diagnosis.

Treatment

Topical steroids and cycloplegics or periocular steroid injections can be used when ocular inflammation is confined to the anterior segment. If there is posterior segment involvement in BD, systemic therapy is required. The choice of medications is determined by the severity of the disease. In general the treatment of the ocular form of the disease must be more aggressive when the patient has complete BD with neurologic and vascular involvement, multiple recurrences of uveitis, male sex, bilateral involvement, origin in the Mediterranean area or Far East.[16] The most commonly used anti-inflammatory drugs are corticosteroids, cytotoxic agents, cyclosporine, and colchicine.

Corticosteroids

Systemic corticosteroids have a rapid and definite anti-inflammatory effect in all phases of ocular BD, but especially in the acute phase. However, these drugs failed to prevent visual deterioration and the ultimate blindness from the consequences of ocular BD. [6,7,26] Still, steroid therapy — oral (1-1.5 mg/kg/day), intravenous (1 gr/day for 3 days) or both — forms an important component in the plan of care for the patients with BD. In posterior segment inflammation, oral corticosteroids are used in combination with immunosuppressive drugs, and then the steroids are gradually tapered. The advantage of this regimen is to obtain benefit from the immediate corticosteroid anti-inflammatory action while waiting for the full effect of the cytotoxic drug's action, which usually takes 3 to 6 weeks. In chronic cases, maintenance doses (15-30 mg/day) of prednisone may be required in combination with immunosuppressives.

Chlorambucil [Leukeran]

Chlorambucil was the first cytotoxic drug to be used in the care of patients with ocular BD and it is still commonly used as the most efficacious single agent. The mode of action of this slow-acting alkylating agent is similar to that of cyclophosphamide. The usual starting dose is 0.1 mg/kg/day. A favorable response may take 1 to 3 months to become evident. Subsequently the drug dose is reduced, and a maintenance dose is given for 1 to 2 years depending on the symptoms, ocular findings, bone marrow tolerance, often special aspects of the individual. Chlorambucil therapy can be complicated by precipitous and persistent pancytopenia, amenorrhea, infection, and secondary malignancy.[27] Malignancy later in life is a significant concern in patients receiving greater than 1300 mg in toto of chlorambucil.[28] Pivetti-Pezzi and associates reported that early intervention with chlorambucil produced a better outcome than did corticosteroid therapy.[29] A high-dose short-term chlorambucil regimen for BD has also produced a favorable outcome.[30] In contrast, Tabbara reported that the long-term results with chlorambucil were not particularly encouraging, with 75 % of eyes having a visual acuity of 20/200 or less when this agent was used as the sole therapy.[31]

Cyclophosphamide [Cytoxan]

Cyclophosphamide has been used widely in Japan with considerable efficacy in preventing the ocular attacks and maintaining good visual acuity for long periods.[32] It has been used successfully in cases refractory to chlorambucil. [7] It is a fast-acting alkylating agent which can be administered orally (1 mg/kg/day) or intravenously (750-1000 mg/m2/day every 4 weeks) with a potential kidney and bladder toxicity.

Azathioprine [Imuran]
Azathioprine is a purine analogue, and it is usually used in combination therapy. Recently it was reported that oral azathioprine (2.5 mg/kg/day) decreased recurrences of ocular BD.[33] We generally use it in combination with cyclosporine and low-dose prednisone.

Cyclosporine
Cyclosporine is not cytotoxic and therefore presumably cannot induce clonal deletion of autoaggressive cells. It is relatively selective in inhibition of T-lymphocytes. In randomized studies, cyclosporine was found more effective for prevention of BD ocular recurrences than was colchicine and cyclophosphamide.[34, 35] In a study done by Nussenblat et al, cyclosporine was found to be effective in ocular BD, but the dose employed (10 mg/kg/day) was associated with significant renal toxicity.[36] A recent study from Turkey suggested an initial dose of 5 mg/kg/day cyclosporine be used in the treatment of ocular BD, and if the intraocular inflammation does not totally resolve at this dosage or if the inflammatory process recurs, a combination of the cyclosporine with low doses of steroid should be considered.[37] Cyclosporine therapy is generally limited to bilateral sight-threatening cases of BD. Serum creatinine and creatinine clearance must be followed closely. It should be noted that abrupt discontinuation may lead to "rebound" phenomenon. As mentioned above, our bias here, if cyclosporine or Imuran are to be used, is to use them together, along with prednisone, in a manner similar to solid organ transplant rejection prevention therapy.

Tacrolimus [FK 506]
Tacrolimus (FK 506) is a newly developed immunosuppressive drug with an immunologic activity very similar to cyclosporin. It binds to alpha 1 acid glycoprotein in serum and selectively inhibits CD 4+ T-lymphocytes. Japanese FK 506 Study Group on Refractory Uveitis reported favorable effects in 75% of 53 patients with refractory uveitis, including 41 with BD. [38] Recently, subcutaneous interferon alpha was successfully used in patients with mucocutaneous disease and ocular involvement.[39, 40]

Plasmapheresis
Plasmapheresis induces rapid remission but does not prevent relapse or change the final outcome of the ocular inflammation.[41] There are also reports on **pentoxifylline [Trental]**[42] and **thalidomide** [43] used in the care of patients with BD.

Eye Surgery
Surgery is indicated whenever visual improvement can be expected and the eye has been free of inflammation for a minimum of 3 months.

Operating on eyes with cataract and uveitis has been previously reviewed by Foster and associates.[44] Their recommendations for a successful cataract surgery and for minimizing the postoperative uveitis are as follows:

> Uveitis should be inactive for at least 3 months preoperatively, systemic and topical steroids should be used prophylactically for 1 week preoperatively and continued post-operatively, immunosuppressive drugs should be continued, complete removal of cortical material should take place, and one-piece PMMA posterior chamber intraocular lens should be used if the patient and the surgeon understand the special nature of this surgery, its risks, and the prognosis for success.

> Laser photocoagulation in some patients is indicated, primarily to forestall vitreous hemorrhage and the development of neovascular glaucoma, as well as to decrease macular edema resulting from vein occlusion. In a study from Turkey it was reported that the photocoagulation therapy for BD was well tolerated and successful in closing retinal capillary non-perfusion areas and eliminating retinal neovascularization.[45]

Prognosis

The systemic prognosis is good in patients with BD in the absence of CNS involvement or involvement of the major vessels...In a study from Lebanon 75% of the patients who were untreated, or treated with steroids, lost vision to no light perception in a mean of 3.5 years.[46] In an Israeli report of patients with ocular BD at 6 to 10 year follow-up, 10% of eyes had visual acuity of 20/40 or better, 16% 20/50 to 20/100, 18% were 20/200 to 20/400, 26% were counting fingers or less, and 30% had no light perception.[47]

In a recent study from Japan, it was reported that despite immunosuppressive therapy, 35% of the patients lost 5 or more lines of visual acuity or became legally blind in 3 years.[48] It was also reported that male sex, posterior segment involvement, and frequent attacks are among the poor prognostic factors.

In a series from the USA, the visual prognosis is better. In a study from our service at Massachusetts Eye and Ear Infirmary, only 2 of 29 (7%) patients and 12 of 58 (21%) eyes had vision of 20/200 or less after a mean follow-up of 4 years (1-8 years).[49] Although not commonly employed in clinical practice for BD, it was suggested that flash electroretinography together with pattern visually evoked potentials were good indicators for visual prognosis as well as for monitoring posterior segment changes. [50]

References

1) Behcet H. Uber rezidivierende, aphthose, durch ein Virus verursachte Geshwure am Munde, am Auge und an den Genitalien. Dematologische Wochenschr 1937;36:1152-1157

2) Levinsky RJ, Lehner T. Circulating immune complexes in Behçet's Syndrome and recurrent oral ulcers. J Lab Clin Med 1981;97:559

3) Mishima S, Masuda K, Izawa Y et al. Behçet's Disease in Japan: ophthalmologic aspects. Trans Am Ophthalmol Soc 1979;77:225-279

4) Yazici H. Behçet's Disease. In Klippel JH, Dieppe PA, editors. Rheumatology, 6.20.1-6.20.6, London 1994, Mosby

5) O'Duffy JD. Behçet's Disease. In Kelley WN, Harris ED Jr, Ruddy S, Sledge CB (eds). Textbook of Rheumatology, Philadelphia, WB Saunders, 1985, pp 1174-1178

6) Chajec T, Farinaru M. Behcet's Disease: Report of 41 cases and a review of the literature. Medicine 1975;54:179

7) Baer JC, Raizman MB, Foster CS. Ocular Behçet's Disease in the United States. Clinical presentation and visual outcome in 29 patients. In Masahiko U, Shigeaki O, Koki A (eds). Proceedings of the Fifth International Symposium on the Immunology and Immunopathology of the Eye, Tokyo, 13-15 March 1990. New York, Elsevier Science, 1990, p383

8) Ammann AJ, Johnson A, Fyfe GA, et al. Behcet' Syndrome. J Pediatr 1985;107:41

9) Ohno S, Aoki K, Sugiura S, et al. HLA-B5 and Behçet's Disease. Lancet 1973

10) Yazici H, Chamberlain MA, Schieuder I, et al. HLA antigens in Behçet's Disease. A reappraisal by a comparative study of Turkish and British patients. Ann Rheum Dis 1980;39:344-348

11) Mizushima Y, Inaba G, Mimura Y, et al. Guide for diagnosis of Behçet's Disease, report of Behçet's Disease Research Committee, Japan, 1987, Ministry of Health and Welfare

12) International Study Group for Behçet's Disease. Criteria for diagnosis of Behçet's Disease. Lancet 1990;335:1078-1080

13) Nakae K, Masaki F, HashimotoT, et al. A nationwide epidemiological survey on Behçet's Disease, report 2: association of HLA-B51 with clinic-epidemiological features, report of Behçet's Disease Research Committee, Japan, 1992, Ministry of Health and Welfare, pp 70-82

14) Ersoy F, Berkel, A, Firat T, et al. HLA antigens associated with Behçet's Disease. In Dausset J, Suejgaard A, (eds): HLA and disease, 100, Paris, 1976, PUB

15) Koc Y, Gullu I, Akpek G, et al. Vascular involvement in Behçet's Disease. J Rheumatol 1992;19:402-410

16) Mishima S, Masuda S, Izawa Y, et al. Behçet's Disease in Japan: Ophthalmologic aspects. Trans Am Ophthalmol Soc 1979;77:225

17) Cohen S, Kremer I, Tiqva P. Bilateral corneal immune ring opacity in Behçet's Syndrome. Arch Ophthalmol 1991;109:324-325

18) Olivieri I, Genovesi-Ebert F, Signorini G, Pasero G. Conjunctival ulceration in Behçet's Syndrome. Ann Rheum Dis 1992;51(4):574-579

19) Atmaca LS. Fundus changes associated with Behçet's Disease. Graefe's Arch Clin Exp Ophthalmol 1989;227:340-344

20) Hooper PL, Rao NA, Smith RE. Cataract extraction in uveitis patients. Surv Ophthalmol 1990;35:120-144

21) Ciftci OU, Ozdemir O. Cataract extraction comparative study of ocular Behçet's Disease and idiopathic uveitis. Ophthalmologica 1995;209:270-274

22) Jorizzo JL, Solomon AR, Canolli MD, Leshin B. Neutrophilic vascular reactions. J Am Acad Dermatol 1988;43:783

23) Niwa Y, Mizushima Y. Neutrophil-potentiating factors released from stimu

lated lymphocytes: Special reference to the increase in neutrophil-potentiating factors from streptococcus-stimulated lymphocytes of patients with Behçet's Disease. Clin Exp Immunol 1990;79:353

24) Valesini G, Pivetti-Pezzi P, Manstrandea F, et al. Evaluation of T cell subsets in Behçet's Syndrome using anti-T cell monoclonal antibodies. Clin Exp Immunol 1985;60:55-60

25) Al-Dalaan A, Al-Sedairy S, Al-Balaa S, et al. Enhanced interleukin 8 secretion in circulation of patients with Behçet's Disease. J Rheumatol 1995;22:904-907

26) Mamo JG, Bagdasarian A. Behçet's Disease: A report of 28 cases. Arch Ophthalmol 1964;71:38

27) Matteson EL, O'Duffy JD. Treatment of Behçet's Disease with chlorambucil. Proceedings of the International Congress on Behçet's Disease, Rochester, MN, 1989, p575

28) Travis LB, Curtis RE, Stoval M, et al. Risk of leukemia folloving treatment for non-Hodkin's lymphoma. J Natl Cancer Inst 1994;86(19):1450-1457

29) Pivetti-Pezzi P, Gasparri V, De Liso P, et al. Prognosis in Behçet's Disease. Ann Ophthalmol 1985;17:20-28

30) Tessler HH, Jennings T. High-dose short-term chlorambucil for intractable sympathetic ophthalmia and Behçet's Disease. Br J Ophthalmol 1990;74:353-57

31) Tabbara KF. Chlorambucil in Behçet's Disease: A reappraisal. Ophthalmology 1983;45:265-268

32) Hijikata K, Masuda K. Visual prognosis in Behçet's Disease: Effects of cyclophosphamide and colchicine. Jpn J Ophthalmol 1978;16:284-329

33) Yazici H, Pazarli H, Barnes C, et al. A controlled trial of azathioprine in Behçet's Syndrome. N Engl J Med 1990;322:281

34) Masuda K, Nakajima A. Adouble masked study of ciclosporin treatment in Behçet's Disease. In Schindler R, ed. Ciclosporin in autoimmune diseases, Berlin, Springer-Verlag, 1985, pp162-164

35) Ozyazgan Y, Yurdakul S, Yazici H, et al. Low dose cyclosporin A versus pulsed cyclophosphamide in Behçet's Syndrome: A single masked trial, Br J Ophthalmol 1992;76:241-243

36) Nussenblat RB, Palestine AG, Chan CC, et al. Effectiveness of cyclosporine therapy for Behcet's Disease. Arthritis Rheum 1985;28:672

37) Atmaca LS, Batioglu F. The efficacy of cyclosporin A in the treatment of Behçet's Disease. Ophthalmic Surg 1994;25(5):321-327

38) Mochizuki M, Masuda K, Sakane T, et al. A clinical trial of FK 506 in refractory uveitis. Am J Ophthalmol 1993;115:763-769

39) Alpsoy E, Yilmaz E, Basaran E. Interferon therapy for Behçet's Disease. J Am Acad Dermatol 1994;31:617-619

40) Kotter I, Eckstein A, Zierhut M. Therapy of ocular manifestations in Behçet's Disease with interferon alpha. Invest Ophthalmol & Vis Sci 1996;37(3):1036

41) Raizman MB, Foster CS. Plasma exchange in the therapy of Behçet's Disease. Graefe's Arch Clin Exp Ophthalmol 1989;227:360

42) Yasui K, Kobayashi M, et al. Succesful treatment of Behcet's Disease with pentoxifylline. Ann Intern Med 1996;124(10):891-893

43) Gardner-Medvin JM, Smith NJ, Powell RJ. Clinical experience with thalidomide in the management of severe aral and genital ulceration in conditions such as Behcet's disease: use of neurophysiological studies to detect thalodomide neuropathy. Ann Rheum Dis 1994; 53(12)828-832

44) Foster CS, Fong LP, Singh G. Cataract surgery and intraocular lens implantation in patients with uveitis. Ophthalmolgy 1984;96:281

45) Atmaca LS. Experience with photocoagulation in Behçet's Disease. Ophthalmic Surg 1990;21(8):571-576

46) Mamo JG. The rate of visual loss in Behçet's Disease. Arch Ophthalmol 1970;84:451

47) Ben Ezra D, Cohen E. Treatment and visual prognosis in Behçet's disease. Br J Ophthalmol 1986;70:589

48) Sakamato M, Akazamak K, Nishioka Y, et al. Prognostic factors of vision in patients with Behçet's Disease. Ophthalmology 1995;102:317-321

49) Foster CS, Baer JC, Raizman MB. Therapeutic responses to systemic immune suppressive chemotherapy agents in patients with Behçet's Syndrome affecting the eyes. Proceedings of the Fifth International CONGRESS on Behçet's Disease, Rochester, MN, 1989. In O'Duffy JD, Kokmen E (eds):Behçet's Disease; Basic and clinical aspects. New York, M Dekker, 1991, pp581-588

50) Cruz RD, Adachi-Usami E, Kakisu Y. Flash electroretinograms and pattern visually evoked cortical potentials in Behçet's Disease. Jpn J Ophthalmol 1990;34:142-148

Connection Between Arthritis and Ocular Disease
C. Stephen Foster, M.D.

The eye is made up primarily of collagen, as are ligaments, tendons, and tissue within joint spaces. It is, perhaps, primarily because of this similarity in composition that the eye is often affected by many of the same diseases which affect joints. Some of these disorders include Juvenile Rheumatoid Arthritis, Adult Rheumatoid Arthritis, Systemic Lupus Erythematosus, Relapsing Polychondritis, Behçet's Disease, Wegener's Granulomatosis, Polyarteritis Nodosa, and Scleroderma or systemic sclerosis. Additionally, the type of vasculature that is present in the eye has special characteristics that produce an extraordinarily sensitive "barometer" or "sentinel canary" in the eye for potentially lethal vasculitis that can be associated with the aforementioned collagen vascular diseases. Specifically, we know from considerable experience that, despite the fact that a patient's rheumatoid arthritis may be "burned out" as far as active inflammation of the joints in concerned, nonetheless, the patient may well have subclinical rheumatoid vasculitis affecting various internal organ systems. The eye is a very potent indicator of such subclinical potentially lethal vasculitis, and if the eye becomes involved with retinal vasculitis, uveitis, scleritis, or peripheral ulcerative keratitis in such a patient, we take that as a very strong signal that the patient must be evaluated extremely carefully for potentially underlying vasculitis affecting viscera and we also take such a potentially blinding ocular lesion very seriously from the standpoint of the need for aggressive systemic immunomodulatory therapy in order to prevent permanent damage to the eye from such lesions.

For example, we have seen many instances in which patients with systemic lupus erythematosus appear, systemically, to be doing quite well (indeed, the patient's rheumatologist has told her that she is doing very well) despite the fact that new-onset uveitis, scleritis, or retinal vasculitis has developed in one eye. We have seen this story evolve to life-threatening central nervous system vasculitis and/or lupus renal disease when the onset of the ocular inflammation was not taken as an indication for increasing the vigor of systemic therapy. We have tried diligently, therefore, over the past 15 years to raise the consciousness, not only of ophthalmologists worldwide, but also of rheumatologists and other internists of the valuable indicator that the eye can be with respect to seriousness of associated arthritic/collagen vascular disease.

Association of Ocular Inflammatory Disease with Inflammatory Bowel Disease
C. Stephen Foster, M.D.

Even more surprising than the association between arthritis and eye inflammation, at least to some people, is the association between bowel inflammation and eye inflammation. But history tells us that such an association exists. This may be true not only in infectious inflammatory bowel disease, as in the case of Whipple's disease, but also in inflammatory bowel disease generally considered to be autoimmune. For example, approximately 5% of patients who develop ulcerative colitis will experience episodes of recurrent uveitis; some patients with ulcerative colitis will develop other ocular inflammation such as scleritis or episcleritis. And an even greater association exists between Crohn's disease (regional ileitis) and ocular inflammation.

Interestingly, the "activity" of the inflammation in the eye and the inflammation in the gut rarely are concurrent, i.e., the inflammatory bowel disease may be under excellent control, but uveitis may be extremely troublesome; and vice versa, the eye may not have any difficulty at all, while the patient is having major flare-ups of inflammatory bowel disease. Additionally, one of the more effective medications for control of the inflammatory bowel disease activity, Sulfasalazine, has proven to be, in our hands and in those of others, particularly disappointing in controlling the recurrent episodes of uveitis in patients with inflammatory bowel disease-associated uveitis. Patients with IBD-associated uveitis generally required one of the immunomodulatory medications, such as Methotrexate, Azathioprine, or Cyclosporin.

In contrast, patients with "irritable bowel syndrome"- associated uveitis can often be managed with topical therapy or with sulfasalazine or an oral non-steroidal anti-inflammatory agent without the need of a immunosuppressant/immunomodulatory agent. The exact connection between "irritable bowel syndrome" (as opposed to inflammatory bowel disease), and uveitis is not well proven, but it has been the strong clinical impression of many experts of uveitis that such an association exists.

CHAPTER 9

Neurological complications and neuro-Behçet's

Neurological problems are difficult for many Behçet's patients to understand, and can be especially frightening if (or when) these symptoms occur unexpectedly. What could be worse than feeling like you aren't in control of your own body? In the last few years, there have been several large-scale research studies on BD patients with neurological involvement. The good news is that not all neuro symptoms appear to be indicators of serious disease. In addition, the frequency of neurological complications is relatively low compared to some other Behçet's symptoms. As we shall see in an article below, the rate of CNS involvement ranges from 4-49%, but in large-scale studies, the percentage tends to be low: approximately 5% (Siva, 2001).

This chapter will provide information from several different sources: a research study performed by Akman-Demir et al in 1999; an article on neuro-Behçet's by Aksel Siva, M.D. (reprinted with permission); and an excerpt from the description of neuro-Behçet's found in **Behçet's Disease: A Contemporary Synopsis**, edited by Plotkin, Calabro and O'Duffy (also reprinted with permission).

In a comprehensive 1999 research study of 200 Behçet's patients with neuro complications, Akman-Demir et al (1999) separated typical neurological symptoms into two primary categories: those with good vs. poor prognoses.[1]

The following factors appear to indicate a **good overall prognosis** for patients with neuro-BD, providing the ability to live and function independently:
1) a normal CSF (cerebrospinal fluid) result
2) secondary or non-parenchymal involvement (e.g. raised intracranial pressure due to dural sinus thrombosis)
3) less than two acute attacks of neuro symptoms and signs lasting more than 24 hours
4) living independently at the time of hospital admission

The following factors may indicate a **poor prognosis** for neuro-BD patients:
1) abnormal CSF (with elevated protein/cell count)
2) parenchymal involvement (e.g. cognitive impairment, paralysis on one side of the body, behavioral changes and/or sphincter disturbance)

3) two or more attacks of neurological symptoms
4) needing assistance for the activities of daily living
5) a relapse during steroid tapering
6) a progressive course of neurological symptoms over time

Akman-Demir et al also defined the most- and least-common neurologic findings in BD patients with parenchymal problems. The **most common symptoms**, appearing in 50% or more of the parenchymal cases, were: pyramidal signs; paralysis on one side of the body; behavioral changes (apathy and/or disinhibition); sphincter disturbances and/or impotence; and headache. In 10-40% of the cases, the findings were: brainstem signs; pyramidocerebellar syndrome; sensory disturbance; fever; paraperesis; meningeal signs; movement disorders; and excessive daytime sleep. The **least common findings**, appearing in only 5% or less of the cases, were: seizures; psychiatric disturbance (an acute psychotic episode); hearing loss; cerebellar syndrome; optic neuropathy; hemianopia (blindness in half the field of vision in one or both eyes); and aphasia (impairment of speech).

Neuropsychological testing of 74 of the 200 subjects also provided some interesting results. According to Akman-Demir, "the most commonly and most severely affected function was memory processes." There were problems with learning and recall; "attention deficit was the second most common abnormality (60%), but in 55% of these it was mildly impaired..... Orientation, language, arithmetic skills and directed spatial attention functions were all normal." Unfortunately, the neuropsychological deficits tended to increase over time, regardless of the frequency of neurological flare-ups.

Kidd et al (1999) discussed **CSF analysis** as a way to identify cases of neuro-Behçet's.[2] According to Kidd, "Gille and colleagues reported that oligoclonal immunoglobulin bands disappeared from CSF following an acute attack (Gille et al, 1990). This is in stark contrast to multiple sclerosis, in which persistent oligoclonal bands are present in the CSF of 97% of patients (McLean et al, 1990; Zeman et al, 1996)." In Akman-Demir's study of BD patients (above), researchers stated that "oligoclonal IgG bands were present in 16%...one or two persisting bands were found in these latter patients. None of the patients showed more than two bands."[1]

It is possible for Behçet's patients to have **"silent" neurological involvement;** that is, abnormal neuro test results without obvious symptoms, other than possible complaints of headache.[2,3] Researchers are unsure if this silent involvement is self-limited, or if it progresses into more serious levels of neuro-Behçet's. There are several tests available to help physicians determine if their Behçet's patients are experiencing subclinical neurological involvement.

Selected tests for detecting subclinical neurological involvement:

1) SPECT scan: According to Avci et al (1998), "functional imaging using SPECT may detect abnormalities at an initial stage prior to their progression to morphological

damage detectable by MRI, and this imaging modality can be used even in cases which show no neurologic symptoms."[7] Interested readers may also wish to obtain Markus et al's article *rCBF abnormalities detected and sequentially followed by SPECT in neuro-Behçet's syndrome with normal CT and MRI imaging* (J Neurol 1992;239:363-66)

2) P300: According to Kececi and Akyol (2001), P300 testing can be used to reflect subclinical neurological involvement in Behçet's disease. In a research study with fifteen Behçet's patients and fifteen healthy control subjects, "patients had significantly prolonged latencies of P300 as com pared to normal controls, but no significant differences in amplitude. Patients showed a significantly delayed motor response time ...eight of the patients had motor response time values exceeding the mean of controls by two standard deviations."[8]

3) Pupillometric tests: Bayramlar et al (1998) used these tests to check for autonomic nervous system dysfunction in 31 BD patients vs. 41 healthy control subjects. All four tests revealed significant differences between the patients and the controls: mean pupil cycle time (PCT) was 1156 ms for patients, 919 ms for controls; mean dark-adapted pupil size (DAPS) was 0.45 for patients, 0.56 for controls; and both the 0.05% pilocarpine drop test and 1% phenylephrine test showed significant differences in iris sensitivity for both groups. The amount of sensitivity to 0.05% pilocarpine was correlated with the length of the patient's illness.[9]

4) F response parameters: Budak et al (2000) suggest that the F response parameters can be used as a "sensitive method for detection of mild neuropathy in patients with other-wise normal nerve conduction tests...In the tibial nerve, the F response latency and chronodispersion were increased, while F amplitude, duration, and persistence were all decreased in patients with BD... ulnar motor and sensory, tibial motor and sural sensory nerve conduction studies failed to differentiate the patients with BD and controls. In the ulnar nerve, the F response parameters were not significantly different for the populations."[10]

In addition to these tests, the **blink reflex** may help in brainstem evaluation of Behçet's patients. Ortega et al (2001) described a patient who had normal brainstem auditory evoked responses (BAER). Further testing by blink reflex uncovered abnormalities that were later con-firmed by MRI. Follow-up blink reflex studies were normal when the patient was asymptomatic.[11]

Before moving on to Dr. Siva's article below, we will close this section with a final quote from Kidd et al:[2] "The prognosis for recovery following acute [neuro-BD] relapse was in general good, the majority of patients becoming symptom-free. However, of those who were followed-up, 28% underwent further attacks, and 14% became significantly disabled as a consequence of either the absence of recovery or the development of a progressive disease course."

References:

1) Akman-Demir G, Serdaroglu P, Tasci B et al. Clinical patterns of neurological involvement in Behçet's disease: evaluation of 200 patients. Brain 1999;122:2171-2181 2) Kidd D, Steuer A, Denman AM, Rudge P. Neurological complications in Behçet's syndrome. Brain 1999;122:2183-2194
3) Akman-Demir G, Baykan-Kurt B, et al. Seven-year follow-up of neurologic involvement in Behcet syndrome. Arch Neurol 1996 Jul;53(7):691-4
4) Gille M, Sindic CJ, et al. Atteintes neurologiques et la maladie de Behcet. Acta Neurol Belg 1990;90:234-47
5) McLean BN, Luxton RW, Thompson EJ. A study of immunoglobulin G in the cerebrospinal fluid of 1007 patients with suspected neurological disease using isoelectric focusing and the Log IgG-Index. Brain 1990;113:1269-89
6) Zeman AZ, Kidd D, McLean BN, Kelly MA et al. A study of oligoclonal band begative multiple sclerosis. J Neurol Neurosurg Psychiatry 1996;60:27-30
7) Avci O, Kutluay E et al. Subclinical cerebral involvement in Behçet's disease: a SPECT study. Eur J Neurol Jan;5(1):49-53
8) Kececi H, Akyol M. P300 in Behçet's patients without neurological manifestations. Can J Neurol Sci 2001;28:66-69
9) Bayramlar H, Hepsen IF, Uguralp M, Boluk A, Ozcan C. Autonomic nervous system involvement in Behçet's disease: a pupillometric study. J Neuroophthalmol 1998 Sep;18(3):182-6
10) Budak F, Efendi H, Apaydin R, Bilen N, Komsuoglu S. The F response parameters in Behçet's disease. Electromyogr Clin Neurophysiol 2000 Jan-Feb;40(1):45-8
11) Ortega M, Garcia A, Martinez V, Calleja J. Usefulness of the blink reflex in a case of brainstem neuro-Behçet's disease. [Spanish]. Rev Neurol 2001 Jan 1-15;32(1):67-70

The following article by Aksel Siva, M.D. first appeared in **BD News**, August 2001(2): 2, p2. It is reprinted with the permission of Dr. Siva, as well as Hasan Yazici, M.D., Editor of **BD News**.

Neurological Involvement in Behçet's Disease

Aksel Siva, M.D.

One of the many systems to be involved in Behçet's disease (BD) is the nervous system. The reported range for the frequency of neurological involvement has been 2.2%-49%. This rate does not exceed 5% in large series. We have found the mean age of onset for BD and neurologic involvement to be 26.7 +/- 8.0, and 32.0 +/- 8.7 years respectively in our patient population, similar to other reports. Neurological involvement in BD occurs more commonly in males.

Patients with BD may present with different neurological problems, related either directly or indirectly to the disease. Central nervous system (CNS) involvement secondary to vascular inflammation, cerebral venous (dural) sinus thrombosis, the Neuro-Psycho-Behçet variant in which an organic psychotic syndrome is prominent, are direct effects and are designated as "Neuro-Behçet Syndrome" (NBS). Tension-type headache, depression and neurologic complications of BD treatment are among the indirect neuro-psychiatric consequences of the disease. Peripheral nervous system involvement is extremely rare. However, neurophysiological studies may demonstrate non-specific findings in some patients.

Clinical features:

The most common neurological symptom among patients with BD is **headache**. Some patients with BD report a paroxysmal migraine-like pain, which is bilateral, frontal, of moderate severity, and throbbing. This type of headache generally starts after the onset of the systemic findings of BD, and may be seen during exacerbations of systemic findings, such as oral ulcerations or skin lesions, though this is not always the rule. This non-structural headache of BD commonly is not associated with primary neurological involvement. However, a substantial number of patients with BD may report a severe headache of recent onset, not consistent with a co-existing primary headache or ocular inflammatory pain. These patients require further evaluation even if they do not have neurological signs, as this headache may indicate the onset of NBS. *[JZ: An interesting 2001 study by Bahra et al added to the headache literature: According to their report, the PET scan on a migraine patient "provided evidence that migraine [without aura] involves the brainstem." Although this test was not specifically performed on a Behçet's patient, one cannot underestimate the importance of brainstem involvement in neuro-Behçet's cases. More information on this study can be found in the following reference: Bahra A et al.* **Brainstem activation specific to migraine headache.** *Lancet 2001 Mar 31; 357(9261): 1016-7.]*

In addition to headache alone, NBS may present with focal or multifocal **CNS dysfunction** with or without headache. The most common symptoms detected at onset in patients with BD besides headache are: weakness on one side of the body (hemiparesis) or both legs (paraparesis); brainstem and cerebellar symptoms such as double vision, dysarthria [difficulty speaking, due to impairment of the tongue or other muscles essential to speech], facial weakness, tremor and gait instability; and to a lesser extent cognitive and behavioral symptoms. Rare presentations include isolated optic neuritis, psychiatric manifestations referred to as Neuro-Psycho-Behçet Syndrome, epilepsy, aseptic meningitis, intracerebral hemorrhage due to ruptured aneurysms, extrapyramidal syndromes [causing involuntary movements and changes in muscle tone and in posture], and peripheral neuropathy.

Clinical and neuro-imaging evidence confirm that NBS can present with a variety of neurological symptoms, and display findings which may be subclassified in two major forms. One is due to small vein disease and causes the focal or multifocal CNS involvement manifested in the majority of patients (CNS-NBS, or intra-axial NBS). The second form is due to cerebral venous sinus thrombosis (CVT or extra-axial NBS), which has more limited symptoms, a better prognosis, and generally an uncomplicated outcome. Some authors consider to designate only CNS parenchymal involvement as NBS, and include cerebral venous sinus thrombosis within the spectrum of so-called vasculo-Behcet. However, as both have neurological consequences, we favor to identify them as "intra-axial NBS" and "extra-axial NBS," respectively. These two types of involvement occur in the same individual very rarely. We have not observed such a combination in our patient population. These two forms of NBS presumably have a different pathogenesis. Many CNS-NBS patients with small vessel inflammation have a relapsing-remitting course initially, with some ultimately developing a secondary progressive course later. A few CNS-NBS patients will have a progressive CNS dysfunction from the onset. Patients with CVT are more likely to experience a single uncomplicated episode, and rarely further episodes of intracranial hypertension.

As patients with CNS-NBS are young and present with an acute or subacute brainstem syndrome [causing double vision, vertigo, nausea, and/or vomiting] or a hemiparesis [one-sided paralysis], their disease may be mistaken for multiple sclerosis or stroke of young onset, especially in the absence of the systemic signs and symptoms of BD. Notably, we have observed that in most cases with BD who present with neurological manifestations, a careful history will reveal either the presence or a past history of recurrent oral ulcerations with or without other systemic findings of the disease. Furthermore, neuro-imaging is highly suggestive of NBS.

Neuro-imaging:

Neuro-imaging studies in CNS-NBS have shown that cranial magnetic resonance imaging (MRI) is both specific and more sensitive than computerized tomography [CT] in demonstration of the typical reversible inflammatory parenchymal lesions. Lesions are generally located within the brainstem, occasionally with extension to the diencephalon, and basal ganglia at the base of the cerebral hemispheres. Hemispheric lesions within the periventricular and subcortical white matter are not common. MRI/MR-venography is highly sensitive in demonstrating CVT.

Cerebrospinal Fluid (CSF):

If performed during the acute stage, CSF studies usually show inflammatory changes (i.e. increased cells and an elevated level of protein) in most cases of CNS-NBS. CSF in patients with CVT may be under increased pressure, but the cellular and chemical composition is usually normal. An inflammatory CSF usually indicates a bad prognosis.

Treatment:

Neurological involvement in BD is heterogeneous and it is difficult to predict its course, prognosis, and response to treatment. Acute attacks of CNS-Neuro-Behcet syndrome are treated with either oral prednisolone (1 mg/kg for two weeks) or with high dose intravenous methylprednisolone (IVMP 1 g/day) for 5-7 days. Both should be followed with oral tapering over two to three months in order to prevent early relapses. Colchicine, azathioprine, cyclosporine A, cyclophosphamide, methotrexate, chlorambucil, immuno-modulatory agents such as interferon-alpha and, more recently thalidomide, have been shown to be effective in treating some of the systemic manifestations of BD, but none of these agents have been shown beneficial in CNS-NBS in a properly designed study. Cyclosporine was reported to cause neuro-toxicity or to accelerate the development of CNS symptoms, and therefore its use in NBS is not recommended. Cerebral venous sinus thrombosis in BD is treated with a short course of steroids, sometimes with the addition of anticoagulation. Long-term prophylactic treatment is not warranted in these patients, as recurrences are uncommon.

References from Dr. Siva's article appear on page 136.

Neuro-Behçet's Syndrome

Robert S. Lesser and Raphael J. DeHoratius

Central nervous system (CNS) involvement in Behçet's disease (BD) is one of the most serious complications of this illness. Much of the literature supports neuro-Behçet's Syndrome (NBS) as having a variable and often poor prognosis with only the administration of immunosuppressive agents offering some clinical benefit. The diagnosis is frequently difficult to establish and is usually entertained after a thorough laboratory evaluation has excluded other more common infectious and noninfectious etiologies of nervous system pathology. Notwithstanding these qualifications and under the appropriate clinical setting, a thorough history and physical examination remain the sine qua non in arriving at the correct diagnosis of NBS.

Clinical Presentation

Although Behçet's disease may affect all parts of the neuraxis with multiple lesions occurring simultaneously, the following three patterns were proposed to characterize **the various forms of NBS**: [2]

> 1) A brainstem syndrome, which may be either episodic or progressive. Cranial nerve palsies *[JZ: disorders of any of the 12 cranial nerves, which control the following senses:*
>
> | | |
> |---|---|
> | *I* | *Smell* |
> | *II* | *Vision* |
> | *III* | *Eye movements: up/down/inward* |
> | *IV* | *Eye movements: downward/inward* |
> | *V* | *Facial sensation and movement (this is the trigeminal nerve)* |
> | *VI* | *Lateral (sideways) eye movement* |

VII   *Facial movement*
VIII   *Hearing and balance*
IX   *Throat function (determines hoarse ness of voice,swallowing ability)*
X   *Swallowing and heart rate*
XI   *Neck and upper back movement*
XII   *Tongue movement]*

diplopia [double vision], nystagmus [constant, involuntary, cyclical movement of the eyeball], dysarthria [difficulty speaking, due to impairment of the tongue or other muscles essential to speech], ataxia [defective muscular coordination, especially voluntary muscular movements], limb weakness, and pyramidal signs [eg. muscle weakness, problems with reflexes] may be present.[2,5,13]

2) A <u>meningomyelitic syndrome</u> characterized by paraplegia [paralysis of lower portion of the body and legs] or quadriplegia [paralysis of all four limbs and trunk], headache, fever, nuchal rigidity [stiff neck], and cerebrospinal fluid (CSF) pleocytosis [an increase in the number of lymphocytes in the CSF]. In addition, recurrent episodes of culture-negative meningitis, encephalitis, and transient or terminal brainstem signs [causing double vision, vertigo, nausea, and/or vomiting] may occur in this subset of patients.[2,5,13]

3) <u>Organic confusional syndrome</u>, which may be transient, or progressive to dementia.[2,5] Other investigators have characterized a wide spectrum of psychological and mental symptoms and signs including memory impairment, character disorders, apathy, lethargy, altered consciousness, disorientation, insomnia, delirium, euphoria, psychomotor agitation, depression, emotional lability [mood swings], hallucinosis, paranoid attitudes, anxiety, suicidal ideation, delusions and hypochondriasis [abnormal anxiety about one's health]. [11,13,30,38]

Complicating the clinical picture of NBS is the occurrence of these three patterns of neurological complications in various combinations.[5,13] Additional reports have expanded the original neurological observations to include the simultaneous occurrence of motor and sensory symptoms and signs; papilledema [swelling and inflammation of the optic nerve] resulting either from active uveitis or benign intracranial hypertension (pseudotumor cerebri), the latter of which may be secondary to cerebral venous sinus thrombosis [CVT]; Bell's palsy [one-sided facial paralysis]; palatal myoclonus [spasms/contractions of one or both sides of the roof of the mouth]; spinal cord and spinal and peripheral nerve lesions with manifestations including the Brown-Sequard syndrome [weakness on one side of the body, and loss of pain/temperature sensation on the other], cauda equina syndrome [when an inflamed spinal column compresses nerves extending below the spinal cord - resulting problems include impotence, urinary incontinence at night, diminished sensation in bladder and rectum, and loss of reflexes in the ankle], and peripheral neuropathy; cerebellar signs including nystagmus [constant, involuntary eyeball movements], tremor, and ataxia [problems with muscular coordination]; pyramidal tract syndrome with Babinski's sign, clonus [spasms of muscular contraction and relaxation], spastic paralysis, and altered speech; extrapyramidal signs [can include tremors, involuntary twitching of limb or facial muscles, and Parkinsonian movements]; mixed pyramidal and extrapyramidal features; transient ischemic attacks ["mini-strokes"]; hemiparesis or quadriparesis; Weber's syndrome; bulbar paralysis; pseudobulbar palsy; paralysis of bladder and bowel; focal or generalized seizures; aphasia [impaired ability to communicate]; dysphagia [difficulty in swallowing]; hyperesthesia [increased sensitivity to pain or touch]; coma; and subarachnoid and intracranial hemorrhages.[5-14,16-18,20,41] Signs of spinal cord involvement, besides including the Brown-Sequard syndrome, may consist of depressed sensations below a certain dermatome [specific sections of the skin receiving nerve sensations from various spinal cord segments], hyperactive patellar [knee] reflexes, absent lower abdominal reflexes, and paralysis of the bladder with urinary retention.[30]

Hearing impairment and vertigo secondary to cochlear and vestibular abnormalities, respectively, have been reported in Behcet's disease. Although this inner-ear involvement is a late complication, it tends to progress during the ensuing years. Although the episodes of vertigo may become more frequent, they may decrease in duration and intensity.[28] The autonomic nervous system may also be affected in BD with reduction of the sympathetic excitability at the level of the hypothalamus, and enhancement of peripheral parasympathetic reactivity including the presence of a cholinomimetic pupil.[36,39] Dilsen [40] has shown significant hyperactivity of the peripheral sympathetic system in BD.

In a series of 31 patients with NBS, the symptoms and signs in order of decreasing frequency were:

> increased tendon reflexes
> spastic paresis [muscular rigidity accompanying partial paralysis]
> headache
> sensory impairment
> extensor plantar reflexes [extension of the big toe in an abnormal response when the lateral sole of the foot is stroked from heel to toe]
> ankle clonus [alternating, spasmodic, muscle contraction and relaxation]
> absent abdominal reflexes [contraction of abdominal wall muscles when overlying skin is stimulated]
> dysarthria [speech impairment]
> difficulty in urination and defecation

nystagmus [constant involuntary eyeball movement]
diplopia [double vision]
facial nerve palsy [paralysis]
coordination difficulties
dysphagia [difficulty in swallowing, or inability to swallow]
focal convulsions [seizures]
vertigo
impaired visual acuity [loss of sharpness of vision].[13]

In another series, the most common clinical picture of NBS was transient or persistent episodes of brainstem dysfunction. [20]

Epidemiology, Clinical Correlates, and Histopathology
Central nervous system involvement affects approximately 4 to 42% of patients suffering from BD, and the onset of the neurological symptoms occurs from 1 to 11 years after the initial presentation of the triple symptom complex. [9,13,20] The mean age of the onset of CNS involvement is in the fourth decade, and the natural history of NBS is noteworthy for both spontaneous remissions and exacerbations. [9,31]

However, ***three distinct clinical patterns of NBS have been recently described; these have consisted of***

[1] exacerbations and remissions
[2] transition into a chronic progressive stage after a phase of exacerbations and remissions
[3] a chronic progressive course from the onset. [37]

The mortality associated with NBS has ranged from 47 to 66%;[2] however, more recently, Hughes [20] and Kalbian [7] have reported a more favorable outcome in their series of patients with various neurological deficits.

Pathologically, the CNS lesions may be distributed diffusely; a review of the autopsy literature has shown involvement of cerebral gray and white matter, hippocampus, basal ganglia, optic nerves, internal capsule, midbrain, pons, cerebellum, medulla, and spinal cord. [4,13,21,29,32-35,42] Histopathological examination has been remarkable for lymphocytic meningeal infiltration, scattered small necrotic or softened foci in the white matter, perivascular lymphocytic cuffing, especially around venules, and diffuse axonal demyelination and degeneration. [4,13] Swelling of the neuronal cells and the presence of pontine multinucleated nerve cells have been observed on tissue section. [13] Essentially, most authorities have viewed vasculitis as the main underlying pathogenic mechanism to explain the nervous system complications of BD, with thrombophlebitis contributing to certain manifestations, such as pseudotumor cerebri. [2,6,9,13,20]

The **electroencephalographic tracings** of patients with NBS have ranged from normal results to those demonstrating diffuse alpha-wave patterns and mild to moderate increases of diffuse slow waves (slow alpha and theta). The EEG patterns have often correlated with the clinical signs and underlying brain pathology, and the presence of diffuse alpha waves may be dependent upon the preserved functioning of the brainstem reticular-activating system. [50]

Selected References:
2) Pallis CA, Fudge BJ. The neurological complications of Behçet's syndrome. Arch Neurol Psychiat 1956;75:1-14

4) McMenemey WH, Lawrence BJ. Encephalomyelopathy in Behçet's disease. Report of necropsy in two cases. Lancet 1957;2:353-58

5) Strachan RW, Wigzell FW. Polyarthritis in Behçet's multiple symptom complex. Ann Rheum Dis 1963;22:26-35

6) Wolf SM, Schotland DL, Phillips LL. Involvement of nervous system in Behçet's syndrome. Arch Neurol 1965;12:315-25

7) Kalbian VV, Challis MT. Behçet's disease. Report of twelve cases with three manifesting as papilledema. Am J Med 1970;49:823-29

8) O'Diffy JD, Carney JA, Deodhar S. Behçet's disease: report of 10 cases, 3 with new manifestations. Ann Int Med 1971;75:561-70

9) Chajek T, Fainaru M. Behçet's disease. Report of 41 cases and a review of the literature. Medicine 1975;54:179-96

10) O'Duffy JD, Goldstein NP. Neurological involvement in seven patients with Behçet's disease. Am J Med 1976;61:170-78

11) Kozin F, Haughton V, Bernhard GC. Neuro-Behcet disease: two cases and neuroradiologic findings. Neurology 1977;27:1148-1152

12) Wright VA, Chamberlain MA. Behçet's syndrome. Bull Rheum Dis 1978-9;29:972-77

13) Shimizu T, Ehrlich GE, Inaba G, Hayashi K. Behcet disease (Behcet syndrome). Semin Arthritis Rheum 1979;8:223-60

14) Pamir MN, Kansu T, Erbengi A, Zileli T. Papilledema in Behçet's syndrome. Arch Neurol 1981;38:643-5

16) Harper CM, O'Neill BP, O'Duffy JD, Forbes GS. Intracranial hypertension in Behçet's disease: demo;nstration of sinus occlusion with the use of digital subtraction angiography. Mayo Clin Proc 1985;60:419-22

17) Wechsler B, Bousser MG, Huong Du LT, et al. Central venous sinus thrombosis in Behçet's disease (letter). Mayo Clin Proc 1985;60:419-22

18) Shuttleworth EC, Voto S, Sahar D. Palatal myoclonus in Behçet's disease. Arch intern Med 1985;145:949-50

20) Hughes RAC, Lehner T. Neurological aspects of Behçet's syndrome. In Lehner T, Barnes CG, eds: Behçet's Syndrome. Clinical and Immunological Features. Proceedings of a Conference Sponsored by the Royal Society of Medicine, February 1979. London, Academic Press, 1979:241-258

21) Rubinstein LJ, Urich H. Meningo-encephalitis of Behçet's disease: Case report with pathological findings. Brain 1963;86:151-160

28) Brauma I, Fainaru M. Inner ear involvement in Behçet's disease. Arch Otolaryngol 1980;106:215-17

29) Katoh K, Matsunaga K, Ishigatsubo Y, et al. Pathologically defined neuro-, vasculo-, entero-Behçet's disease. J Rheumatol 1985;12:1186-1190

30) Mavioglu H. Behçet's recurrent disease. Analytical review of the literature. Mo Med 1958;55:1209-1222

31) Alema G, Bignami A. Involvement of the nervous system in Behçet's disease. In Monacelli M, Nazzaro P, eds: Behçet's Disease. International Symposium on Behçet's Disease, Rome, 1964. Basel, S Karger, 1966:52-66

32) Normal RM, Campbell AMG. The neuropathology of Behçet's disease. In Monacelli M, Nazzaro P, eds: Behçet's Disease. International Symposium on

Behçet's Disease, Rome, 1964. Basel, S Karger, 1966:67-78

33) Fukuda Y, Hayashi H, Kuwabara N. Pathological studies on neuro-Behçet's disease. In Inaba G, ed: Behçet's Disease. Pathogenetic Mechanism and Clinical Future. Proceedings of the International Conference on Behçet's Disease, October 23-24, 1981, Tokyo. Tokyo University Press, 1982127-143

34) Totsuka S, Hattori T, Yazaki M, Nagao K. Clinicopathology of neuro-Behçet's disease. In Inaba G, ed: Behçet's Disease. Pathogenetic Mechanism and Clinical Future. Proceedings of the International Conference on Behçet's Disease, October 23-24, 1981, Tokyo. Tokyo University Press, 1982:183-196

35) Hayashi H, Fukuda Y, Kuwabara N. Pathological studies on neuro-Behçet's disease: With special reference to leukocytic reaction. In Inaba G, ed: Behçet'sDisease. Pathogenetic Mechanism and Clinical Future. Proceedings of the International Conference on Behçet's Disease, October 23-24, 1981, Tokyo. Tokyo University

36) Sugiura S, Ohno S, Ohguchi M, et al. Autonomic nervous system in Behçet's disease. In Inaba G, ed: Behçet's Disease. Pathogenetic Mechanism and Clinical Future. Proceedings of the International Conference on Behçet's Disease, October 23-24, 1981, Tokyo. Tokyo University Press, 1982:81-88

38) Siva A, Ozdogan H, Yazici H, et al. The neurological and psychiatric complications of Behçet's disease and neuro-CT findings (abstract 61). Royal Society of Medicine international conference on Behçet's disease, Sept 5 and 6, 1985, London, England

39) Tabuchi S, Ishikawa S. Pupillary study of Behçet's disease (abstract 65). Royal Society of Medicine international conference on Behçet's disease, Sept 5 and 6, 1985, London, England

40) Dilsen G. Autonomic nervous system in Behçet's disease (abstract 66). Royal Society of Medicine international conference on Behçet's disease, Sept 5 and 6, 1985, London, England

41) Nagata K. Recurrent intracranial hemorrhage in Behcet disease (letter). J Neurol Neurosurg Psychiatry 1985;48:190-1

42) Lakhanpal S, Tani K, Lie JT et al. Pathologic features of Behçet's syndrome: A review of Japanese autopsy registry data. Hum Pathol 1985;16:790-795

50) Matsumoto K, Matsumoto H, Morofushi K. The clinicoelectroencephalographical correlation to the underlying neuropathology in neuro-Behçet's syndrome. In Inaba G, ed: Behçet's Disease. Pathogenetic Mechanism and Clinical Future. Proceedings of the International Conference on Behçet's Disease, October 23-24, 1981, Tokyo. Tokyo University Press, 1982:219-31

Selected References: (from Dr. Siva's article, pp 128-131)

1) Siva A, Fresko I. Behçet's Disease. Curr Treat Options Neurol 2000; 2:435-47

2) Siva A, Kantarci OH, Saip S, Altintas A, Hamuryudan V, Islak C, Kocer N, Yazici H. Behçet's disease: diagnostic and prognostic aspects of neurological involvement. J Neurol 2001: 248:95-103

3) Akman-Demir G, Serdaroglu P, Tasci B. Clinical patterns of neurological involvement in Behçet's Disease: evaluation of 200 patients. Brain 1999; 122:2171-81.

4) Kidd D, Steuer A, Denman AM, Rudge P. Neurological complications in Behçet's Syndrome. Brain 1999; 122:2183-94.

5) Wechsler B, Vidailhet M, Bousser MG, Dell Isola B, Bletry O, Godeau P. Cerebral venous sinus thrombosis in Behçet's disease: Long-term follow-up of 25 cases. Neurology 1992; 42:614-18

6) Kocear N, Islak C, Siva A, Saip S, Akman C, Kantarci O, Hamuryudan V. CNS involvement in neuro-Behçet's syndrome: a MR study. AJNR 1999; 20:1015-24

CHAPTER 10

Fibromyalgia and Behçet's disease

Fibromyalgia (also known as fibrositis and fibromyositis) creates musculo-skeletal pain, tenderness or stiffness. Some areas of the body that can be affected include the neck, back, elbows, shoulders, chest wall, and knees. Previous (non-Behçet's) studies have shown that the pain of fibromyalgia can become worse in cold and damp weather, through over-exertion, and as a result of emotional stress.[1]

 While a quick computer search uncovered over 1300 studies that have been done on fibromyalgia, only one study in the medical literature specifically looks at the relationship between fibromyalgia and Behçet's disease.[2] In 1998, Yavuz questioned 108 Behçet's patients about their fibromyalgia-type symptoms, and compared the survey results with three control groups: a group of systemic lupus erythematosus (SLE) patients; a group of rheumatoid arthritis (RA) patients; and a group of healthy control subjects. Ten of the 108 Behçet's patients (9.2%) met the American College of Rheumatology criteria for fibromyalgia, and of the 10 patients, 9 were women (90%). The frequency of fibromyalgia in Behçet's patients was higher than the frequency in healthy control subjects, although the results weren't statistically significant. However, while SLE and RA patients with severe symptoms have a higher chance of developing fibromyalgia, this connection doesn't hold true with Behçet's patients: a severe case of Behçet's does not mean that the patient will eventually develop fibromyalgia.

> The following overview of fibromyalgia was written by Robert Bennett, M.D., of Oregon Health Sciences University, and is reprinted with his permission from the Oregon Fibromyalgia website at www.myalgia.com.

Introduction to Fibromyalgia Syndrome
Robert M. Bennet, M.D.

Fibromyalgia (fi-bro-my-AL-ja) syndrome (FMS) is a very common condition of widespread muscular pain and fatigue. Seven to ten million Americans suffer from FMS. It affects women much more than men in an approximate ratio of 20:1. It is seen in all age groups from young children through old age, although in most patients the problem begins during their 20s or 30s. Recent studies have shown that fibromyalgia syndrome occurs world-wide and has no specific ethnic predisposition.

The Symptoms of Fibromyalgia Syndrome

Fibromyalgia syndrome patients have widespread body pain which arises from their muscles. Some FMS patients feel their pain originates in their joints. Pain that emanates from the joints is called arthritis. Extensive studies have shown FMS patients do not have arthritis. Although many fibromyalgia syndrome patients are aware of pain when they are resting, it is most noticeable when they use their muscles, particularly with repetitive activities. Their discomfort can be so severe it may significantly limit their ability to lead a full life. Patients can find themselves unable to work in their chosen professions and may have difficulty performing everyday tasks. As a consequence of muscle pain, many FMS patients severely limit their activities including exercise routines. This results in their becoming physically unfit - which eventually makes their fibromyalgia syndrome symptoms worse.

In addition to widespread pain, other common symptoms include a decreased sense of energy, disturbances of sleep, and varying degrees of anxiety and depression related to patients' changed physical status. Furthermore, certain other medical conditions are commonly associated with fibromyalgia, such as: tension headaches, migraine, irritable bowel syndrome, irritable bladder syndrome, premenstrual tension syndrome, cold intolerance and restless leg syndrome. This combination of pain and multiple other symptoms often leads doctors to pursue an extensive course of investigations - which are nearly always normal.

Diagnosing Fibromyalgia Syndrome

There are no blood tests or x-rays which show abnormalities diagnostic of FMS. This initially led many doctors to consider the problems suffered by FMS patients were all "in their heads" or that fibromyalgia syndrome patients had a form of masked depression or hypochondriasis. *[JZ: Even now, medical papers are still being published that discuss this philosophy. For example, in March 2001, we were treated to "**Fibromyalgia: reality or fantasy?**"[3]]*

Extensive psychological tests have shown these impressions were unfounded. A physician's diagnosis of FMS is based on taking a careful history and the finding of tender areas in specific areas of muscle. These locations are called "tender points" or "trigger points." They are tender to palpation and often feel somewhat hardened if the muscle is stroked. Frequently, pressure over one of these areas will cause pain in a more peripheral distribution, hence the term trigger point.

The Long Term Outcome for Fibromyalgia Syndrome

Musculoskeletal pain and fatigue experienced by fibromyalgia syndrome patients is a chronic problem which tends to have a waxing and waning intensity. There is currently no generally accepted cure for this condition. According to recent research, most patients can expect to have this problem lifelong. However, worthwhile improvement may be obtained with appropriate treatment, as will be discussed later. There is often concern on the part of patients, and sometimes physicians, that

FMS is the early phase of some more severe disease, such as multiple sclerosis, systemic lupus erythematosus, etc. Long term follow-up of fibromyalgia patients has shown that it is very unusual for them to develop another rheumatic disease or neurological condition. However, it is quite common for patients with "well established" rheumatic diseases, such as rheumatoid arthritis, systemic lupus and Sjogren's syndrome to also have fibromyalgia. It is important for their doctor[s] to realize they have such a combination of problems, as specific therapy for rheumatoid arthritis and lupus, etc. does not have any effect on FMS symptoms. Patients with fibromyalgia syndrome do not become crippled with the condition, nor is there any evidence it effects the duration of their expected life span. Nevertheless, due to varying levels of pain and fatigue, there is an inevitable contraction of social, vocational and avocational activities which leads to a reduced quality of life. As with many chronic diseases, the extent to which patients succumb to the various effects of pain and fatigue are dependent upon numerous factors, in particular their psycho-social support, financial status, childhood experiences, sense of humor, and determination to push on.

The Treatment of Fibromyalgia Syndrome

The treatment of FMS is frustrating for both patients and their physicians. In general, drugs used to treat musculoskeletal pain, such as aspirin, non-steroidals and cortisone, are not particularly helpful in this situation. As in any chronic pain condition, education is an essential component that helps patients understand what can or can't be done, as well as teaching them to help themselves. It is important for a patient's physician to discover whether there is a cause for sleep disturbances. Such sleep problems include sleep apnea, restless leg syndrome and teeth grinding. If the cause for a patient's sleep disturbance cannot be determined, low doses of an anti-depressive group of drugs, called tricyclic anti-depressants, may be beneficial. Patients need to understand these medications are not sleeping pills and are not addictive when used in low dosages (e.g., Amitriptyline 10 mg at night) and have very few side effects. In general, routine use of sleeping pills such as Halcion, Restoril, Valium, etc. should be avoided as they impair the quality of deep sleep. A [more recent] hypnotic medication, Ambien, is claimed to avoid this problem.

There is increasing evidence that a regular exercise routine is essential for all fibromyalgia syndrome patients. This is easier said than done because increased pain and fatigue caused by repetitive exertion makes regular exercise quite difficult. However, those patients who do get into an exercise regimen experience worthwhile improvement and are reluctant to give up. In general, FMS patients must avoid impact loading exertion such as jogging, basketball, aerobics, etc. Regular walking, the use of a stationary exercycle and pool therapy utilizing an Aqua Jogger (a flotation device which allows the user to walk or run in the swimming pool while remaining upright) seem to be the most suitable activities for FMS patients to pursue. Supervision by a physical therapist or exercise physiologist is of benefit wherever possible. In general, 20 minutes of physical activity, 3 times a week at 70% of maximum heart rate (220 minus your age) is sufficient to maintain a reasonable level of aerobic fitness.

Drugs such as aspirin and Advil are not particularly effective and seldom do more than take the edge off FMS pain. In general, narcotic pain killers containing codeine and other similar substances should be avoided, as in the long run they down regulate the body's production of its own pain produced substances called endorphins. Particularly painful areas often may be helped for a short time (2-3 months) by trigger point injections. This involves injecting a trigger point with a local anesthetic (usually 1% Procaine) and then stretching the involved muscle with a technique called spray and stretch. It should be noted the injection of a tender point is quite painful (indeed, if it is not painful the injection is seldom successful). After the injection, there is typically a 2-4 day lag before any beneficial effects are noted. Other techniques which directly help the tender areas on a transient basis are heat, massage, gentle stretching and acupuncture.

About 20% of FMS patients have a co-existing depression or anxiety state which needs to be appropriately treated with therapeutic doses of anti-depressants or anti-anxiety drugs often in conjunction with the help of a clinical psychologist or psychiatrist. Basically, patients who have a concomitant psychiatric problem have a double burden to bear. They will find it easier to cope with their FMS if the psychiatric condition is appropriately treated. It is important to understand fibromyalgia syndrome itself is not a psychogenic pain problem and that treatment of any underlying psychological problems does not cure the fibromyalgia. Most FMS patients quickly learn there are certain things they do on a daily basis that seem to make their pain problem worse. These actions usually involve the repetitive use of muscles or prolonged tensing of a muscle, such as the muscles of the upper back while looking at a computer screen. Careful detective work is required by the patient to note these associations and where possible to modify or eliminate them. Pacing of activities is important; we have recommended patients use a stop watch that beeps every 20 minutes. Whatever they are doing at that time should be stopped and a minute should be taken to do something else. For instance, if they are sitting down, they should get up and walk around or vice versa. Patients who are involved in fairly vigorous manual occupations often need to have their work environment modified and may need to be retrained in a completely different job. Certain people are so severely affected that consideration must be given to some form of monetary disability assistance. This decision requires careful consideration, as disability usually causes adverse financial consequences as well as a loss of self-esteem. In general, doctors are reluctant to declare fibromyalgia patients disabled and most FMS applicants are automatically turned down by the Social Security Administration. However, each patient needs to be evaluated on an individual basis before any recommendations for or against disability are made.

Support Groups and Doctors Interested in FMS

It is not always easy to find a doctor who has an interest in treating FMS patients. If you experience such difficulty, call your local chapter of the Arthritis Foundation or the Fibromyalgia Alliance of America (1-800-717-6711). Meeting other patients with fibromyalgia syndrome, particularly in the context of an educational seminar, is often a benefit in gaining a greater self-understanding. Over the past 5 years, many such support groups have sprouted up in the major cities and even in some of the smaller rural areas. Again, the name and location of such support groups may be found through the local Arthritis Foundation or the Fibromyalgia Alliance of America.

Research into Fibromyalgia Syndrome

Over the past 10 years there has been increasing recognition and interest in fibromyalgia syndrome. There are now over 1,000 publications in medical literature relating to this condition. The National Institutes of Health has recently recognized the importance of fibromyalgia as a cause of musculoskeletal pain and has set aside specific funding for research in this area. *[JZ- Interested readers may want to visit a medical library to read two specific issues of* **Current Rheumatology Reports**. *The first, published in April 2001 (Vol 3, No. 2), has a large section devoted to fibromyalgia, including information on the following topics: cognitive dysfunction in fibromyalgia; the role of gender; exercise for FM patients (risks vs. benefits); complementary and alternative therapies for FM; the role of psychiatric disorders; fibromylagia and other unexplained clinical conditions; juvenile primary fibromyalgia syndrome; and a report on clinical drug trials.*

The most recent issue (Vol 4, No. 4; 2002), also has an extensive fibromyalgia section, edited by Robert M. Bennett, M.D., who provided the fibromyalgia chapter for this book. This **Current Rheumatology Reports** *section has articles on the following topics: managing fibromyalgia patients; fibromyalgia and association with silicon breast-implant rupture; neural mechanisms that generate FM pain; adult growth hormone deficiency in patients with FM; and information on recent clinical trials.]*

[JZ: Additional information on FM treatment:

Recent studies have looked at the use of Navoban (tropisetron) in treating symptoms of fibromyalgia.[4,5] Haus et al (2000) found that a daily dose of 5mg tropisetron provided a significant reduction in patients' pain after ten days' use, with benefits continuing to increase during the remaining 18 days of the study. In addition to pain reduction, patients also experienced less depression, anxiety, sleep disturbances and dizziness. Gastrointestinal problems and headaches were the most commonly reported side effects of using this drug.

Other studies - with varying success rates - suggest the use of nutritional supplementation,[6] magnetic fields,[7] ascorbigen,[8] chiropractic manipulation,[9] copper wire bed sheets,[10] and acupuncture[11] to reduce the symptoms of fibromyalgia.]

References

1) Yunus MB, Masi AT, Calabro JJ, et al. Primary fibromyalgia (fibrositis): clinical study of 50 patients with matched normal controls. Semi Arthritis Rheum 1981; 11:151-171

2) Yavuz S, Fresko I, Hamuryudan V, Yurdakul S, Yazici H. Fibromyalgia in Behçet's syndrome. J Rheumatol 1998 Nov;25(11):2219-20

3) Olin R. [Fibromyalgia — fantasy or reality?]. Lakartidningen. 2001 Mar 21;98(12):1437, 1439.

4) Haus U et al. Oral treatment of fibromyalgia with tropisetron given over 28 days: influence on functional and vegetative symptoms, psychometric parameters and pain. Scand J Rheumatol Suppl. 2000;113:55-8.

5) Papadopoulos IA et al. Treatment of fibromyalgia with tropisetron, a 5HT3 serotonin antagonist: a pilot study. Clin Rheumatol. 2000;19(1):6-8.

6) Merchant RE, Andre CA. A review of recent clinical trials of the nutritional supplement Chlorella pyrenoidosa in the treatment of fibromyalgia, hypertension, and ulcerative colitis. Altern Ther Health Med. 2001 May-Jun;7(3):79-91.

7) Alfano AP et al. Static magnetic fields for treatment of fibromyalgia: a random ized controlled trial. J Altern Complement Med. 2001 Feb;7(1):53-64.

8) Bramwell B et al. The use of ascorbigen in the treatment of fibromyalgia patients: a preliminary trial. Altern Med Rev. 2000 Oct;5(5):455-62.

9) Hains G, Hains F. A combined ischemic compression and spinal manipulation inthe treatment of fibromyalgia: a preliminary estimate of dose and efficacy. J Manipulative Physiol Ther. 2000 May;23(4):225-30.

10) Biasi G et al. A new approach to the treatment of fibromyalgia syndrome. The use of Telo Cypro]. Minerva Med. 1999 Jan-Feb;90(1-2):39-43. Italian.

11) Berman BM et al. Is acupuncture effective in the treatment of fibromyalgia? J Fam Pract. 1999 Mar;48(3):213-8. Review.

CHAPTER 11

Information on peripheral neuropathy

Do you feel pain, tingling and/or numbness in your arms, legs, hands or feet? Is there weakness or a feeling of "heaviness" in your limbs? If so, you may have peripheral neuropathy (PN). While the central nervous system complications of Behçet's disease have been well documented, very little research has been done on peripheral nerve involvement in BD. As a result, many health care professionals feel there is no connection, and may downplay these symptoms during office visits. There are so many anecdotal accounts of Behçet's patients complaining of PN symptoms, however, that a brief overview is warranted.

Three research studies conducted in 1980, 1995 and 1999[1,2,3] discussed peripheral nerve involvement in the small number of Behçet's patients enrolled in their studies. In each case, approximately 25% of the participants exhibited some signs of peripheral neuropathy. Budak et al (2000) studied Behçet's patients who had no clinical signs of neuro-BD, and had otherwise normal nerve conduction tests.[4] They discovered that only the F response parameters were sensitive enough to detect the presence of Behçet's-related neuropathy, and that - if it occurred at all - peripheral neuropathy was most prevalent in the legs and feet of Behçet's patients. The challenge comes in determining the true cause of a BD patient's peripheral neuropathy. While PN can be directly Behçet's-related, Tattevin et al (1999) explain that some drugs used to treat Behçet's disease may also cause symptoms of PN.[5] Relevant examples include colchicine, which can create a temporary peripheral neuropathy that is reversible by stopping the drug; and Thalidomide, which can cause an irreversible peripheral neuropathy. As a result of this serious potential side effect, the use of Thalidomide requires a baseline nerve conduction test prior to the start of treatment, and follow-up tests every three to six months to determine the extent of any new peripheral nerve involvement before it becomes problematic.

The following information on peripheral neuropathy has been reprinted with the permission of the Neuropathy Association, and is an excerpt from the booklet *Explaining Peripheral Neuropathy*, by Mary Ann Donovan and Norman Latov, M.D., Ph.D. The full booklet can be obtained through the Neuropathy Association's web site at www.neuropathy.org, or by contacting the Association at 60 East 42 Street, Ste 942, New York, NY 10165. Their phone number is 1-800-247-6968.

What is Peripheral Neuropathy?

Peripheral neuropathy is the term used to describe disorders resulting from injury to the peripheral nerves. It can be caused by diseases that affect only the peripheral nerves, or by conditions that affect other parts of the body as well. Symptoms almost always involve weakness, numbness or pain — usually in the arms and legs. The peripheral nervous system is one of the two main divisions of the body's nervous system. (The other is the central nervous system, which includes the brain and spinal cord.) "Peripheral" means away from the center. The peripheral nervous system contains the nerves that connect the central nervous system to the muscles, skin and internal organs.

Three Kinds of Nerves

There are three distinct kinds of nerves: motor, sensory, and autonomic.

Motor nerves are responsible for voluntary movement. Their cell bodies lie within the spinal cord, and their processes transmit signals outward to specialized motor receptors on the skeletal muscles. When you reach to open a door or run to catch a train, for instance, your motor nerves are at work.

Sensory nerves allow us to feel pain, vibrations or touch, to recognize shapes by feel, and to sense where our limbs are positioned in space. Their cell bodies are grouped in specialized structures called sensory "ganglia" next to the spinal cord. They transmit signals from sensory receptors in the skin and other organs, inward to the central nervous system.

Autonomic nerves control involuntary functions like breathing, heartbeat, blood pressure, digestion and sexual function. They work automatically when we're awake or asleep, and are not under our control. Their cell bodies, clustered in autonomic ganglia, are spread throughout the body.

Although most neuropathies affect all three types of nerve fibers to varying degrees, some diseases involve only one or two, and are thus said to be purely or predominantly motor, sensory, or autonomic neuropathies.

Is it Mono- or Polyneuropathy?

A disorder of a single peripheral nerve is called _mononeuropathy_. It is usually caused by trauma, local compression (the nerve is being squeezed), or by inflammation. Examples include Carpal Tunnel Syndrome, which is a wrist and hand disorder, and Bell's Palsy, which is a facial nerve disorder. They affect single nerve trunks in distinct areas.

If there is a problem in two or more nerve trunks in separate areas, and it is caused by a generalized disorder like diabetes, for instance, the neuropathy is then called _mononeuritis multiplex_.

Polyneuropathy, the umbrella name for the greatest number of peripheral neuropathies, means that the disorder is diffuse and symmetric — relatively the same on both sides of the body. When motor and sensory fibers are affected, the neuropathy is called "sensorimotor." It usually begins in the hands and feet — the "distal" ends of the longest nerves.

Neuritis is an inflammation of the nerves caused by infection or the immune system.

What are your symptoms?

Some neuropathies come on suddenly, while others gradually appear over many years. The symptoms depend on the types of nerves affected and their location, but the problem usually starts with weakness, numbness or pain. Here are some of the telltale signs that people describe:

Weakness in the arms or legs

Usually caused by damage to the motor nerves, leg symptoms include difficulty walking or running, "heaviness" — it takes most of your strength just to climb the stairs — and stumbling or tiring easily. Muscle cramps may be common. Neuropathy in the arms may cause difficulties with carrying a load of groceries, opening jars, turning door knobs, or combing your hair. Or you may be frustrated to find you keep dropping things that you thought you had a good grip on.

Numbness, tingling and pain

The sensory nerves, when damaged, can cause many different symptoms. Early on, you may have spontaneous sensations called paresthesias, which include numbness, tingling, pins and needles, prickling, burning, cold, pinching, sharp deep stabbing pains, electric shocks, or buzzing. They are usually worse at night, and are often painful and severe. Unpleasant abnormal sensations brought on by touching or other stimuli are called dyesthesias. Or instead, you may have _anesthesia_, a lessening or absence of sensation, which can cause you to burn or cut yourself and not know it.

Absence of position sense

When you have this symptom, you're probably not sure just where your feet are, and may thus be uncoordinated and unsteady when you walk. Or you may realize that the way you walk has changed, but not be sure exactly how or why. Chances are that you have widened your gait in an unconscious effort to keep your balance, or you may tend to drag your feet.

"Glove and Stocking Sensation"

This is what doctors call the odd feeling you may have that you're wearing stockings or gloves or slippers, when, in fact, your hands and feet are completely bare.

Symptoms of autonomic damage

Damage to the autonomic nerves can cause dizziness when standing up, constipation, diarrhea, sexual dysfunction, and thinning of the skin, with easy bruisability and poor healing.

How is Peripheral Neuropathy treated?

The goals of treatment are twofold:

(1) to eliminate the cause of the disease and

(2) to relieve its symptoms.

Treatment of the underlying condition depends on the cause. [If your neuropathy is caused by autoimmune diseases], these diseases are frequently treated by plasmaphoresis or immuno-suppression, using corticosteroids, intravenous gammaglobulins, or chemotherapy. The pain of neuropathy can be alleviated with medications. Physical therapy and prosthetic devices, if necessary, can help maintain strength and improve walking.

Depending on the cause, therapy can slow, halt or reverse the neuropathy. Once the damage is stopped, the nerves can then regenerate. The extent of recovery depends on how much damage was done. The less the damage, the better the recovery. Therefore, it is very important to diagnose the disease as early as possible and begin therapy.

> The following information on opioid drugs, non-opioid drugs, and topical medications is from the book *Numb Toes and Aching Soles: Coping with Peripheral Neuropathy*, copyright 1999 by John A. Senneff, and is reprinted with permission of the author.

There are several non-opioid drugs that can be used to treat peripheral neuropathy:

For burning pains

    (a) all of the so-called tricyclic antidepressants, including Elavil (amitriptyline) (this one particularly where sleep disorders are a problem); Norpramin (desipramine); Pamelor (nortriptyline); and Tofranil (imipramine).

    (b) Mexitil (mexiletine hydrochloride)

    (c) Neurontin (gabapentin)

    (d) Ultram (tramadol)

For shooting, stabbing, or "electric shock" pains

    (a) Dilantin (phenytoin)

    (b) Klonopin (clonazepan)

    (c) Neurontin (gabapentin)

    (d) Tegretol (carbamazepine)

For aching, persistent pains

    (a) Catapres (clonidine)

    (b) Klonopin (clonazepan)

    (c) Lioresal (baclofen) - particularly when accompanied by spasms and cramping

    (d) Neurontin (gabapentin).

General information on opioids for treating pain

Opioids (a.k.a. narcotics) interact with receptors located in the spinal cord and brain, producing euphoria, sedation and analgesia. They alter the mind's perception of painful stimuli by deadening painful impulses transmitted from the peripheral nerves. A significant feature of the analgesia is that it occurs without loss of consciousness.

Many medical professionals are reluctant to prescribe opioids for PN pain, thinking (or at least claiming) them to be largely ineffective for that purpose. Still, for numerous PN sufferers, they seem to provide the only relief available when pain becomes really overpowering. (This is sometimes referred to as "breakthrough pain" because it seems to break through or overwhelm relief provided by regular medication.)

Opioids are chemically related to morphine. Commonly prescribed formulations include morphine itself, codeine, Dilaudid (hydromorphone), Demerol (meperidine), Dolophine (methadone), Sublimaze (fentanyl), OxyContin (oxycodone) and MS Contin (morphine sulfate).

Often there is a choice as to how opioids will be given. Orally, by pill or liquid, is usually preferred because of cost and convenience. Injections when called for may be either into a vein, muscle, over the spinal cord, or under the skin. Injections produce a quicker result and reduce the amount of opioids required to achieve an analgesic effect. Implanted pumps are also used occasionally. Sublimaze is frequently administered by skin patch (Duragesic) for around-the-clock medication.

Occasionally, the drugs listed above, as well as several other opioids, are used in combination with non-opioid analgesics for PN pain. Included are acetaminophen/oxycodone (trade name Percocet), acetaminophen/propoxyphene napsylate (Darvocet), acetaminophen/hydrocodone bitartrate (Vicodin), acetaminophen/codeine (Tylenol 2, 3, 4), aspirin/oxycodone hydrochloride and oxycodone terephthalate (Percodan).

Often a patient is started on one of these combinations, and then if the maximum acceptable ingestion of the non-opioid component is reached before adequate pain relief is obtained, he or she is switched to the straight opioid component.

Respiratory depression, which is a decrease in the number of breaths or the depth of breathing, can occur from morphine and other opioid analgesics. Other possible side effects are constipation, nausea and confusion, any of which can significantly interfere with a person's daily life.

*[In addition to the opioids and non-opioids, **topical medications** can also be used to treat the symptoms of peripheral neuropathy.]*

The principal topical agent being used is capsaicin, a medication derived from cayenne/red peppers... Capsaicin is delivered either in the form of a cream (trade names Zostrix-0.025% capsaicin; Zostrix HP-0.075%; Axsain-0.075%) or lotion (Capsin -0.025%)... These products, which do not require prescriptions, are generally applied three to four times daily to the feet or other affected areas. An initial burning sensation is usually experienced during the first several days. Continued applications over several weeks are recommended for full results to be obtained.

Another topical application sometimes used for neuropathic pain is **EMLA**, a mixture of two local anesthetics — lidocaine (2.5%) and prilocaine (2.5%) — combined in a cream. This medication may be useful if the burning action of capsaicin can't be tolerated.

*The above information was excerpted from the book **Numb Toes and Aching Soles**, which also contains extensive information on alternative therapies to treat peripheral neuropathy; nutritional supplements and herbal treatments; experimental or "unapproved" drugs; and other (more standard) medical therapies. It is available at bookstores, through amazon.com, or through the publisher at **www.medpress.com**.*

References

1) Kidd D et al. Neurological complications in Behcet's syndrome. Brain 1999 Nov;122 (Pt 11):2183-94

2) Mateos-Colino A et al. Neuro-Behcet: a follow-up of 4 cases treated with chlorambucil. An Med Interna 1995 Dec;12(12):600-2

3) Afifi AK et al. The myopathology of Behcet's disease—a histochemical, light-, and electron-microscopic study. J Neurol Sci 1980 Dec;48(3):333-42

4) Budak et al. The F Response Parameters in Behçet's Disease, Electromyogr Clin Neurophysiol 2000 Jan-Feb;40(1):45-8

5) Tattevin P et al. Neuromuscular complications of long-term treatment of inflammatory diseases. 3 cases. Ann Med Interne (Paris) 1999 Dec;150(8):594-7

CHAPTER 12

Spirituality and health

Do you believe that prayer can influence your health? If so, you're not alone. A 1996 *Time Magazine* survey showed that 82% of Americans believe in the healing power of prayer.[1] A subsequent research report followed trends in alternative medicine use in the U.S. from 1990-1997 (Eisenberg et al, 1998), and found that 35% of the people surveyed had used prayer to address their own health-related problems.[2]

In June 2000, the *Annals of Internal Medicine* published a review of all research studies that had focused on the issue of "Distant Healing" (Astin et al). For the purposes of the study, "distant healing" was defined as the use of "spiritual healing, prayer, and their various [forms]" in ways that create a "conscious, dedicated act of [mental effort], attempting to benefit another person's physical or emotional well-being at a distance."[3] The researchers found over 100 studies that investigated distant healing, but only 23 studies met their strict scientific criteria for inclusion in their review. Of those 23 studies, five specifically dealt with prayer, with a total of 1,489 enrolled patients. 1,383 of these subjects were coronary care patients who were enrolled in two specific studies. Each patient in the coronary "treatment" groups received standard medical treatment plus intercessory Christian prayer (praying for the well-being of others), while each patient in the coronary "control" groups received the usual medical care, without any intercessory prayer. The results? In one study, "the treatment group required less ventilatory support and treatment with antibiotics or diuretics." In the other coronary care study, there were "significant treatment effects on the...coronary care unit score" for the patients who received prayer. None of the patients knew whether or not s/he was in the prayed-for group.

When Astin, Harkness and Ernst looked closely at the results of all 23 research studies mentioned above (which included such "distant healing" practices as "noncontact therapeutic touch," described in 11 of the 23 studies), they found that 13 of the 23 studies (57%) showed statistically significant treatment effects of prayer on the patients' health.

So what do all of these statistics mean for you? That it's quite possible for prayer and other methods of "distant healing" to affect your health in a positive way. As Elisabeth Targ concluded in her 1997 article on "prayer and intentionality" :

> "No experiment can prove or disprove the existence of God, but if in fact [mental] intentions can be shown to facilitate healing at a distance, this would clearly imply that human beings are more connected to each other and more responsible to each other than previously believed."[4]

Readers may be interested in obtaining the following resources, suggested by **Clinician's Guide to Spirituality**, White and Mac-Dougall. McGraw-Hill Medical Publishing Division, c 2001, p9-10:

> Comstock GW, Partridge KB. **Church attendance and health**. Journal of Chronic Diseases; 1972;25:665-672
>
> Strawbridge WJ et al. **Frequent attendance at religious services and mortality over 28 years**. American Journal of Public Health; June 1997;(87):6, 957-61
>
> Koenig HG, Cohen HJ, et al. **Attendance at religious services, Interleukin-6, and other biological indicators of immune function in older adults**. Intl J of Psychiatry in Med. 1997;27:233-50
>
> Byrd RB. **Positive therapeutic effects of intercessory prayer in a coronary care unit population**. Southern Med Journal; 1988;(81):826-29
>
> Oxman TE, Freeman H, Manheimer ED. **Lack of social participation or religious strength and comfort as risk factors for death after cardiac surgery in the elderly**. Psychosomatic Medicine; 1995;57:5-15
>
> Matthews DA, Larson DB, Barry CP. **The Faith Factor: An Annotated Bibliography of Clinical Research on Spiritual Subjects**, Vol 1. John Templeton Foundation, 1994
>
> Matthews DA, Clark C. **The Faith Factor, Proof of the Healing Power of Prayer**. Penguin Books, NY, c1998
>
> Benson H. **Timeless Healing**. Scribner, New York, c1996

References

1) Wallis C. Faith and healing: can prayer, faith and spirituality really improve your physical health? A growing and surprising body of scientific evidence says they can. Time 1996;147:58

2) Eisenberg DM et al. Trends in alternative medicine use in the United States, 1990-1997: results of a follow-up national survey. JAMA. 1998;280:1569-75

3) Astin JA, Harkness E, Ernst E. The efficacy of "distant healing": A systematic review of randomized trials. Ann Intern Med 2000;132:903-910

4) Targ E, Thomson KS. Can prayer and intentionality be researched? Should they be? Altern Ther Health Med. 1997;3:92-6

APPENDIX

Suggested readings on herbal and alternative treatments

The following reference books may be helpful if you are considering the use of herbal products to enhance your health, or to expand your treatment options. A very short list of medical journal articles that specifically addresses alternative treatments for Behçet's has been included. However, general descriptions of alternative programs such as holistic or ayurvedic medicines, special diets, aromatherapy, shiatsu, special diets, and acupuncture, are not addressed here — with one exception: A recent letter by Murray and Aboteen in the ***British Journal of Ophthalmology*** (2002;86:476-477) mentions the case of a man with Behçet's who underwent **acupuncture** to treat "tennis elbow." Two days after his treatment, he developed red areas on his arm that corresponded with the placement of the acupuncture needles. On close examination, these red areas were found to be pustules similar to those created in positive pathergy tests in Behçet's disease. The authors caution that "patients with Behçet's disease should be made aware of this potential complication if they intend to undergo acupuncture."

Please keep in mind that the use of herbs may not be for everyone. It can be easy to think of these products as "natural," and therefore harmless. However, some herbal medicines can interact badly with prescription or over-the-counter (OTC) drugs that you may be taking, and some herbs or supplements could also make your current symptoms worse. **It's extremely important that you let your physician(s) know if you are taking any herbal medicines or supplements prior to undergoing surgery, or starting other treatments.**

Just as you should understand the potential side effects of any new medications before you start taking them, you should also take the time to learn about possible problems or drug interactions with any natural treatments that you're considering. Please don't begin using any herbal products, vitamin supplements, or alternative therapies without first consulting your health care provider.

Books for health care practitioners, or research-oriented patients:

The Complete German Commission E Monographs : Therapeutic Guide to Herbal Medicines, by Mark Blumenthal, Integrated Medicine Communications, c. 1999, ISBN: 0967077273 **Note:** This book is expensive ($165 on the internet, although used copies may be found for much less).

Another book on the subject by the same author costs considerably less — $35 at amazon.com — and is called **Herbal Medicine: Expanded Commission E Monographs.** According to a review from amazon.com's web site: "I get a different dosage recommendation on every bottle and from every so-called herbalist I meet. This is because the FDA does not require studies to be done on herbs and supplements in the US. Thus, we can only turn to what Germany has been doing for over 20 years to study these wonderful plants, because Germany does require that their use, dosage information and side effects be studied before they can be given to the public."

Evidencebased Herbal Medicine, by Irwin, MD Ziment, Michael, Ph.D. Rotblatt, Lippincott Williams & Wilkins Publishers; c.2001, ISBN: 1560534478

The Scientific Validation of Herbal Medicine by Daniel B. Mowrey. NTC Publ, Rev. 1990, ISBN: 0879835346

Botanical Influences on Illness: A Sourcebook of Clinical Research by Werbach and Murray, Third Line Pr, 2nd Ed 2000, ISBN: 1891710001

Herbal Medicines for Neuropsychiatric Diseases: Current Developments and Research by Shigenobu MD, PhD, Kanba et al. Brunner/Mazel, c. 1999, ISBN: 0876308043

Herb Contraindications And Drug Interactions, Second Edition, by Brinker, Stodart (Ed.), Brinker, Eclectic Medical Publications, c. 1998, ISBN: 1888483067

Interactions Between Drugs & Natural Medicines by Chris Meletis, Thad Jacobs. Eclectic Medical Publications, c. 1999, ISBN: 1888483105

General patient and consumer-oriented books:

The Encyclopedia of Popular Herbs: From the Herb Research Foundation, Your Complete Guide to the Leading Medicinal Plants, by McCaleb, Leigh, Morien, Smith (illus), Prima Publishing, c. 2000, ISBN: 076151600X

Herb Contraindications And Drug Interactions, Second Edition, by Brinker, Stodart (Ed.), Brinker, Eclectic Medical Publications, c. 1998, ISBN: 1888483067

Natural Health Complete Guide to Safe Herbs: What Every Consumer Should Know About Interactions and Side Effects for Hundreds of Herbs, Drugs, Supplements, and Foods by Chris D. Melitis, et al. DK Publishing; to be published Dec 2001, ISBN: 0789480735

The New Healing Herbs : The Classic Guide to Nature's Best Medicines Featuring the Top 100 Time-Tested Herbs by Michael Castleman, Rodale, c. 2001, ISBN: 1579543049

The Complete Medicinal Herbal, by Penelope Ody, DK Publishing, c.1993, ISBN: 156458187X

The Complete Illustrated Holistic Herbal : A Safe and Practical Guide to Making and Using Herbal Remedies, by David Hoffman, Element, c. 1996, ISBN: 1852307587

The Way of Herbs : Fully Updated With the Latest Developments in Herbal

Science by Michael Tierra, Pocket Books; 2nd Ed 1998, ISBN: 0671023276

A Field Guide to Medicinal Plants and Herbs of Eastern and Central North America (Peterson Field Guides) by Steven Foster, James A. Duke, Houghton Mifflin Co (Pap); 2nd Ed 2000, ISBN: 0395988144

Encyclopedia of Medicinal Plants, by Andrew Chevallier, DK Publishing, 2nd Ed 2000

The Practice of Chinese Medicine : The Treatment of Diseases With Acupuncture and Chinese Herbs by Maciocia and Macviocia. Churchill Livingstone, c 1997 ISBN: 0443043051

The Pharmacology of Chinese Herbs by Kee Chang Huang, W. Michael Williams. CRC Press, 2nd Ed. 1998, ISBN: 0849316650

Between Heaven and Earth : A Guide to Chinese Medicine by Harriet Beinfield, Efrem Korngold. Ballantine Books, 1992. ISBN: 0345379748

Chinese Herbal Medicine : Formulas and Strategies (Tr. from Chinese/ With Resource Guide to Prepared Medicines Supplement to Chinese Herbal Medicine) by Bensky and Barolet. Eastland Press, c. 1990, ISBN: 0939616106

Medical journal articles about treatment of Behçet's with herbal and alternative methods:

Yu P, Bai H, Zhang W, Wu G. *Effects of acupuncture on humoral immunologic function and trace elements in 20 cases of Behcet's disease.* J Tradit Chin Med. 2001 Jun;21(2):100-2

De Miguel E, Balsa A, Perez de Ayala C, Gijon J. *[Acupuncture in Behcet's syndrome]* Med Clin (Barc). 1987 Apr 4;88(13):564-5. Spanish.

Wu ZW, Yang CY, Bian TY. *Behcet's disease: clinical report of 88 cases treated with herbal decoctions.* J Tradit Chin Med. 1983 Sep;3(3):223-6

Medical journal articles about treatment of rheumatic diseases with alternative medicines:

Ernst E. *Complementary and alternative medicine for pain management in rheumatic diseases.* Curr Opin Rheumatol 2002 Jan;14(1):58-62

Kolasinski SL. *Complementary and alternative therapies for rheumatic disease.* Hosp Pract (Off Ed) 2001 Apr 15;36(4):31-36

Ernst E. *Usage of complementary therapies in rheumatology.* Clin Rheumatol 1998;17(4):301-5

Ernst E. *Evidence-based complementary medicine: A contradiction in terms?* Ann Rheum Dis 1999;58:69-70 (February)

A sampling of cautionary articles from medical research journals:

Murray PI, Aboteen N. *Complication of acupuncture in a patient with Behçet's disease.* British J Ophthalmology 2002;86:476-477. Letter

Tomassoni AJ, Simone K. *Herbal medicines for children: an illusion of safety?* Curr Opin Pediatr. 2001 Apr;13(2):162-9. Review

Borum PR. *Supplements: questions to ask to reduce confusion.* Am J

Appendix 1

Clin Nutr. 2000 Aug; 72(2 Suppl):538S-40S. Review

Huxtable RJ. *The harmful potential of herbal and other plant products*. Drug Saf 1990;5 Suppl 1:126-3

APPENDIX 2

Applying for Social Security
Disability Benefits in the U.S.

*This chapter is a compilation of information from the U.S. Social Security Online web site at **www.ssa.gov**, as well as other sources named throughout the chapter. Most sections are verbatim from the government as part of the public domain. All information is current as of January 2002, but may change at any time due to court rulings or procedural changes. Please check with your local Social Security Office if you have questions on specific benefits. The Social Security Administration may be contacted by calling **1-800-772-1213** between 7 AM and 7 PM, Monday through Friday. People who are deaf or hard of hearing may call the SSA's TTY line at 1-800-325-0778. The SSA's mail address is: Social Security Administration, Office of Public Inquiries, 6401 Security Blvd., Room 4-C-5 Annex, Baltimore, MD 21235-6401. **Local SSA offices** can be found through the toll-free numbers above, or by going to **http://s3abaca.ssa.gov/pro/fol/fol-home.html** .*

As of February 2002, the U.S. Social Security Administration has finally recognized the existence of Behçet's disease as a separate clinical entity: **Behçet's now appears under the "Immune Systems/Inflammatory Arthritis" category of the official SSA *Listing of Impairments*.** This does not mean that Behçet's patients automatically qualify for SSD benefits, as certain medical requirements still need to be met. However, it does mean that patients will no longer have to waste time convincing examiners that BD is worthy of consideration. Specific information on the *Listing of Impairments*, as well as qualifications for Behçet's and other inflammatory, vasculitic and connective tissue diseases, can be found in the shaded section near the end of this chapter.

The most helpful suggestions made by BD patients who have successfully won SSD benefits include:

1) Do not sugarcoat your medical condition, or downplay its effect on your life or your daily activities. Be honest and detailed about your limitations.

2) Psychological problems can be just as incapacitating as physical disabilities. Don't be embarrassed to include them.

3) Many claims are rejected at first — don't give up! According to Charles T. Hall, Esq., Past President of the National Organization of Social Security Claimants' Representatives, (NOSSCR) **only 40% of all disability claims are approved on the first try.**

4) The NOSSCR can provide referrals for lawyers experienced in handling Social Security Disability claims; call 1-800-431-2804, from 9-5 pm EST. Their lawyers receive a percentage of your monetary award if you win, but receive no payment if your claim is denied.

5) If you're currently employed, **remember to check into your company's short-term disability benefits** (if available). You may be eligible to receive some financial benefits before your SSDI payments begin.

6) Keep a copy of all completed forms and documents submitted to Social Security. These copies are most helpful when cases that have been denied are taken before a judge for re-evaluation.

7) If your claim is denied, you have the right to examine your Social Security file, including doctors' reports and other summaries of your case. Note any mistakes that are found, in case they are useful in your appeal.

Disability is a subject that you may read about in the newspaper, but not think of as something that might happen to you. However, the chances of becoming disabled are probably greater than you realize. Studies show that a 20-year-old worker has a 3-in-10 chance of becoming disabled before reaching retirement age.

While we spend a great deal of time working to succeed in our jobs and careers, few of us think about ensuring that we have a safety net to fall back on should we become disabled. This is an area where Social Security can provide valuable help to you.

This chapter will explain the benefits available, how you can qualify, and who can receive benefits on your earnings record. It will also explain how to apply for the benefits and what happens when your application is approved.

How You Qualify for Social Security Disability Benefits

To qualify for benefits, you must first have worked in jobs covered by Social Security. Then you must have a medical condition that meets Social Security's definition of disability. In general, Social Security pays monthly cash benefits to people who are unable to work for a year or more because of a disability. Benefits usually continue until you are able to work again on a regular basis. There are also a number of special rules, called "work incentives," that provide continued benefits and health care coverage to help you make the transition back to work. If you are receiving Social Security disability benefits when you reach age 65, your disability benefits automatically convert to retirement benefits, but the amount remains the same.

How Much Work Do You Need?

In addition to meeting the SSA's definition of disability, you must have worked long enough — and recently enough — under Social Security to qualify for disability benefits. Social Security work credits are based on your total yearly wages or self-employment income. **You can earn up to four credits each year**. The amount needed for a credit changes from year to year. In 2001, for example, **you earn one credit for each $830 of wages or self-employment income**. When you've earned $3,320, you've earned your four credits for the year.

The number of work credits you need to qualify for disability benefits depends on your age when you become disabled. Generally, you need 40 credits, 20 of which were earned in the last 10 years ending with the year you become disabled. However, younger workers may qualify with fewer credits. *Important:* Remember that whatever your age is, you must have earned the required number of work credits within a certain period ending with the time you become disabled. Your Social Security Statement shows whether you meet the work requirement at the time it was prepared. If you stop working under Social Security after the date of the Statement, you may not continue to meet the disability work requirement in the future.

What Social Security Means By "Disability"

The definition of disability under Social Security is different than other programs. Social Security pays only for total disability. No benefits are payable for partial disability or for short-term disability. Disability under Social Security is based on your inability to work. You are considered disabled under Social Security rules if you cannot do work that you did before, and SSA decides that you cannot adjust to other work because of your medical condition(s). Your disability must also last or be expected to last for at least one year, or to result in death.

This is a strict definition of disability. Social Security program rules assume that working families have access to other resources to provide support during periods of short-term disabilities, including workers' compensation, insurance, savings and investments.

How the Social Security System Decides If You Are Disabled

To decide whether you are disabled, there is a step-by-step process involving five questions:

1) Are you working?

If you are working and your earnings average more than $830 a month, you generally cannot be considered disabled. If you are not working, go to the next question.

2) Is your condition "severe"?

Your condition must interfere with basic work-related activities for your claim to be considered. If it does not, they will find that you are not disabled. If your condition does interfere with basic work-related activities, go to the next question.

3) Is your condition found in the list of disabling conditions?

For each of the major body systems, SSA maintains a list of medical conditions that are so severe they automatically mean that you are disabled. (The **Listing of Impairments,** and how to get a copy, is discussed near the end of this chapter.) If your condition is not on the list, they have to decide if it is of equal severity to a medical condition that is on the list. If it is, they will find that you are disabled. If it is not, then go to the next question.

4) Can you do the work you did previously?

If your condition is severe but not at the same or equal level of severity as a medical condition on the list, then they must determine if it interferes with your ability to do the work you did previously. If it does not, your claim will be denied. If it does, proceed to #5.

5) Can you do any other type of work?

If you cannot do the work you did in the past, they see if you are able to adjust to other work. They consider your medical conditions and your age, education, past work experience and any transferable skills you may have. If you cannot adjust to other work, your claim will be approved. If you can adjust to other work, your claim will be denied.

Special Situations

Most people who receive disability benefits are workers who qualify on their own records and meet the work and disability requirements described above. However, there are some situations you may not know about:

Rules For People Who Are Blind: There are special rules for people who are blind or have low vision. You are considered legally blind under Social Security rules if your vision cannot be corrected to better than 20/200 in your better eye, or if your visual field is 20 degrees or less, even with a corrective lens. Many people who meet the legal definition of blindness still have some sight, and may be able to read large print and get around without a cane or a guide dog. If you do not meet the legal definition of blindness, you may still qualify for disability benefits if your vision problems alone, or combined with other health problems, prevent you from working. More information is provided in the booklet, **If You Are Blind Or Have Low Vision-How We Can Help**, available online at the www.ssa.gov web site.

Benefits for Disabled Children: A child under age 18 may be disabled, but the child's disability is not considered when deciding if he or she qualifies for benefits as your dependent. The child's benefits normally stop at age 18 unless he or she is a full-time student in an elementary or high school (benefits can continue until age 19) or is disabled. For a child with a disability to receive benefits on your record after age 18, the following rules apply:

      1) The disabling impairment must have started before age 22, and;
      2) He or she must meet the definition of disability for adults.

Note: An individual may become eligible for a disabled child's benefit from Social Security later in life. For example, a worker may start collecting Social Security retirement benefits at age 62. He has a 38-year old son who has had cerebral palsy since birth. The son will start collecting a disabled "child's" benefit on his father's Social Security record.

How to Put in a Social Security Disability Claim

The Social Security application process is more than just filling in a form. You must first call or visit your local Social Security office and say that you'd like to apply for disability benefits. You will be given an appointment for a phone interview, or a time to meet with a Claims Representative (Disability Examiner) at the SSA office in person. You should request that a copy of the application form be sent to you in advance. Fill it out completely and truthfully. It is illegal to make false statements on this application! Remember to include all physical and/or mental illnesses that have kept you from working: emotional disabilities may be just as incapacitating as physical ones.

You might want to consider getting a copy of the short book, *How to Get SSI & Social Security Disability-An Insider's Step by Step Guide* by Mike Davis (Writers Club Press, c 2001, ISBN 0-595-12574-3) and read it in advance of your interview. There are many excellent suggestions from Mr. Davis (a Disability Examiner himself) in this book, including the following on page 63-64: "The examiner you are contacting is overworked, pressured to move cases, pressured to do quality work, publicly scrutinized via weekly statistics, and has a type A personality (or he wouldn't still be working as a claims examiner)...Much of what the claimant wants to tell the [Disability Examiner] is irrelevant to the claim. Help him get the evidence he needs to make a determination on your case and he will love you....his goal is roughly the same as yours: to complete your claim as accurately and quickly as possible."

Information that Social Security Needs

Claims for disability benefits take more time to process than other types of Social Security claims-from 60 to 90 days. You can help shorten the process by bringing certain documents with you when you apply, and by helping get any other medical evidence you need to show that you are disabled. Here is what you should bring to your meeting:

Information About You:

Your Social Security number and proof of your age

Your original birth and marriage certificates

Names, addresses and phone numbers of doctors, hospitals, clinics and institutions that treated you and the dates of treatment

Names of all medications you are taking

Medical records from your doctors, therapists, hospitals, clinics and caseworkers

Laboratory and test results

A summary of where you worked and the kind of work you did

Your most recent W-2 form, or your tax return if you're self-employed.

Information About Family Members:

Social Security numbers and proof of age for each person applying for benefits

Dates of prior marriages if your spouse is applying

Important: You will need to submit original documents or copies certified by the issuing office. You can mail or bring them to

Social Security. They will make photocopies and return your original documents. If you don't have all the documents you need, don't delay filing for benefits. They will help you get the information you need.

If Your Application Is Denied

After your application has been reviewed and they have looked at the information you have provided, Social Security may decide that you do not meet their qualifications for disability benefits. If you disagree with that decision, you have the right to ask them to look at your application again. The notice you receive from Social Security that says you don't qualify will explain how to make a "reconsideration" request, and the time period in which you must make it. You will need to submit a special "reconsideration" form, not just a written request. If your claim is denied at the reconsideration level, you may then request a hearing before an Administrative Law Judge. It may take anywhere from three months to a year before a hearing can be scheduled.

At any point in this process, you might want to consider hiring an attorney experienced in handling SSD claims, to help you better navigate through the system. The National Organization of Social Security Claimants' Representatives offers a referral service. You can call 1-800-431-2804 during EST business hours to discuss a referral. Typically, an attorney will receive one-quarter of any back benefits that you win, but you will not have to pay him or her if the claim is denied. There is currently a $5300 limit on the amount of money that your attorney may keep from your judgment. *Note:* People who don't have enough work credits to be eligible for Social Security Disability Benefits may possibly qualify for Supplemental Security Income if they have limited income and resources.

When Your Benefits Start

If your application is approved, your first Social Security benefit will be paid for the sixth full month after the date that Social Security says your disability began. For example, if your disability began on June 15, 2001, your first benefit would be paid for the month of December 2001, the sixth full month of disability. Social Security benefits are paid in the month following the month for which they're due. This means that the benefit due for December would be paid to you in January 2002, and so on. In addition, benefits can be retroactive for up to one year of your original application date, if your condition became disabling at least six months prior to the application date.

How Much You Will Receive

The amount of your monthly disability benefit is based on your lifetime average earnings covered by Social Security. The Social Security Statement sent to you each year will tell you how much you would get if you became disabled at the time the Statement was prepared. (If you haven't gotten your Statement, you can complete and transmit the request form online [found at https://s3abaca.ssa.gov/pro/batch-pebes/bp-7004home.shtml].You should receive your statement within 3-4 weeks.)

Medicare Coverage If You're Disabled You are automatically enrolled in Medicare after you get disability benefits for two years. Medicare has

two parts - hospital insurance and medical insurance (Part A and Part B). You only need to pay for Part B coverage. Hospital insurance helps pay for inpatient hospital bills and some follow-up care. The taxes you paid while you were working financed this coverage, so it is free. Medical insurance helps pay doctors' bills, outpatient hospital care and other medical services. You will need to pay a monthly premium for this coverage if you want it. Most people have both parts of Medicare.

Help For Low-Income Medicare Beneficiaries If you get Medicare and have low income and few resources, your state may pay your Medicare premiums and, in some cases, other Medicare costs for which you are normally responsible, such as deductibles and coinsurance. Only your state can decide if you qualify for this assistance. To find out if you do, contact your state or local welfare office or Medicaid agency. For more general information about the program, ask Social Security for the leaflet, *Medicare Savings for Qualified Beneficiaries* (HCFA Publication No.02184).

Taxes On Your Benefits
Some people have to pay federal income taxes on their Social Security benefits. This usually happens only if your total income is high. For example, up to 50 percent of benefits may be taxable for individuals with total income between $25,000 and $34,000; or married couples with total income between $32,000 and $44,000. Up to 85 percent of benefits may be subject to tax for individuals with income over $34,000, or over $44,000 for couples.

At the end of the year, you will receive a Social Security Benefit Statement (Form SSA-1099) that shows the amount of benefits you received. You can use this statement when you are completing your federal income tax return to find out if any of your benefits are subject to tax. If you do have to pay taxes on your Social Security, you may choose to have federal taxes withheld from your benefits.

Your Continuing Eligibility for Benefits
In most cases, you will continue to receive benefits as long as you are disabled. However, there are certain circumstances that may change your continuing eligibility for disability benefits. For example, your health may improve to the point where you are no longer disabled. Or, like many people, you would like to go back to work rather than depend on your disability benefits. There are special rules called "work incentives" that can help you make the transition back to work. These incentives include, but are not limited to, continued monthly benefits and Medicare coverage while you attempt to work on a full-time basis. The law requires that Social Security reviews your case from time to time to verify that you are still disabled. You are told when it is time to review your case, and you are kept informed about your benefit status. You are responsible for letting Social Security know if your health improves or if you go back to work.

Reviewing Your Disability
In general, your benefits will continue as long as you are disabled. However, the law requires that your case is reviewed periodically to see if you are still disabled. How often your case is reviewed depends on whether your condition is expected to improve:

If medical improvement is "**expected**," your case will normally be reviewed within six to 18 months after your benefits start.

If medical improvement is "**possible**," your case will normally be reviewed no sooner than three years.

If medical improvement is "**not expected**," your case will normally be reviewed no sooner than seven years.

What Can Cause Benefits To Stop?

Two things can cause Social Security to decide that you are no longer disabled, and to stop your benefits:

Your benefits will stop if you work at a level that Social Security considers "substantial." Usually, average earnings of $830 or more per month are considered substantial [this amount changes periodically].

Your disability benefits will also stop if Social Security decides that your medical condition has improved to the point that you are no longer disabled. You are responsible for promptly reporting any improvement in your condition, if you return to work, and certain other events (described in a booklet sent to you) as long as you are receiving disability benefits.

Family Benefits

When you start receiving disability benefits, certain members of your family may also qualify for benefits on your record. Each family member may be eligible for a monthly benefit that is up to 50 percent of your disability rate. However, there's a limit to the total amount of money that can be paid to a family on your Social Security record. The limit varies, but is around 150 to 180 percent of your disability benefit.

Benefits For Your Children

When you qualify for Social Security disability benefits, your children may also qualify to receive benefits on your record. Your eligible child can be your biological child, adopted child or stepchild. A dependent grandchild may also qualify. To receive benefits, the child must be unmarried; and

be under age 18; or

be 18-19 years old and a full-time student (no higher than grade 12); or

be 18 or older and have a disability that started before age 22.

Normally, benefits stop when children reach age 18 unless they are disabled. However, if the child is still a full-time student at a secondary (or elementary) school at age 18, benefits will continue until the child graduates or until two months after the child becomes age 19, whichever is first. Within your family, each qualified child may receive a monthly payment up to one-half of your full disability amount, but there is a limit to the amount that can be paid to the family as a whole. This total depends on the amount of your benefit and the number of family members who also qualify on your record. The total varies, but it is approximately 150 to 180 percent of your disability benefit.

Frequently Asked Questions About SSDI

I'm a 30-year-old woman and have been dividing my life between home and periods of work. How much work do I need to make sure I have Social Security disability insurance? This is a good question. Some people don't realize they need recent work under Social Security to qualify for disability benefits. After age 30, you must have 20 credits (5 years) of work in the 10 years before your disability started. Credits are assigned to calendar years based on the amount of your earnings for that year. In 2001, you earn one credit for every $830 in earnings, up to a maximum of four credits for the year (this dollar amount is revised periodically).

If my disability must be expected to last at least a year in order for me to qualify, does this mean I have to wait a year to get benefits? No. You should apply for the benefits as soon as you can. If you are approved, your payments will begin after a 5-month waiting period that starts with the month Social Security decides your disability began.

If I qualify, is there a time limit on how long I can receive disability benefits? No. You will continue to receive your disability benefits as long as your condition keeps you from working. But your case will be reviewed periodically to see if there has been any improvement in your condition and whether you are still eligible for benefits. If you are still disabled when you reach full retirement age, your disability benefit will be automatically converted to a retirement benefit of the same amount.

If I am eligible for Social Security disability benefits, am I also eligible for Medicare benefits? If you receive disability benefits, you become eligible for Medicare 24 months after the date Social Security decides your disability began.

Where can I get a list of the impairments that Social Security considers to be disabling?
"Disability Evaluation Under Social Security" (SSA Pub. No. 64-039) contains the medical criteria that Social Security uses to determine disability. It is intended primarily for physicians and other health professionals. This 205-page book can be obtained free of charge by faxing a request to (410) 965-0696. Impairment listings are also available on the **www.ssa.gov** web site. You can also write or call SSA at: Social Security Administration, Public Information Distribution Center, PO Box 17743, Baltimore, MD 21235-6401. Telephone (410) 965-0945.

Specific Information from the SSA Listing of Impairments relevant to Behçet's disease: Section 14.00: Immune System
(Effective February 19, 2002)

The following sections are applicable to individuals age 18 and over and to children under age 18 where criteria are appropriate.
A. Listed disorders include impairments involving deficiency of one or more components of the immune system (i.e., antibody-producing B cells; a number of different types of cells associated with cell-mediated immunity including T-lymphocytes, macrophages and monocytes; and components of the complement system).

B. Dysregulation of the immune system may result in the development of a connective tissue disorder. Connective tissue disorders include several chronic multisystem disorders that differ in their clinical manifestation, course, and outcome. They generally evolve and persist for months or years, may result in loss of functional abilities, and may require long-term, repeated evaluation and management.

The documentation needed to establish the existence of a connective tissue disorder is medical history, physical examination, selected laboratory studies, medically acceptable imaging techniques and, in some instances, tissue biopsy. However, the Social Security Administration will not purchase diagnostic tests or procedures that may involve significant risk, such as biopsies or angiograms. Generally, the existing medical evidence will contain this information.

A longitudinal clinical record of at least 3 months demonstrating active disease despite prescribed treatment during this period, with the expectation that the disease will remain active for 12 months, is necessary for assessment of severity and duration of impairment.

To permit appropriate application of a listing, the specific diagnostic features that should be documented in the clinical record for each of the disorders are summarized for systemic lupus erythematosus (SLE), systemic vasculitis, systemic sclerosis and scleroderma, polymyositis or dermatomyositis, and undifferentiated connective tissue disorders and the inflammatory arthritides.

In addition to the limitations caused by the connective tissue disorder per se, the chronic adverse effects of treatment (e.g., corticosteroid-related ischemic necrosis of bone) may result in functional loss.

These disorders may preclude performance of any gainful activity by reason of serious loss of function because of disease affecting a single organ or body system, or lesser degrees of functional loss because of disease affecting two or more organs/body systems associated with significant constitutional symptoms and signs of severe fatigue, fever, malaise, weight loss, and joint pain and stiffness. We use the term "severe" in these listings to describe medical severity; the term does not have the same meaning as it does when we use it in connection with a finding at the second step of the sequential evaluation processes in §§ 404.1520, 416.920, and 416.924.

Inflammatory arthritis (14.09) includes a vast array of disorders that differ in cause, course, and outcome. For example, inflammatory spondyloarthropathies include ankylosing spondylitis, Reiter's syndrome and other reactive arthropathies, psoriatic arthropathy, **Behçet's disease**, and Whipple's disease, as well as undifferentiated spondylitis. Inflammatory arthritis of peripheral joints likewise comprises many disorders, including rheumatoid arthritis, Sjögren's syndrome, psoriatic arthritis, crystal deposition disorders, and Lyme disease. Clinically, inflammation of major joints may be the dominant problem causing difficulties with ambulation or fine and gross movements, or the arthritis may involve other joints or cause less restriction of ambulation or other movements but be complicated by extra-articular features that cumulatively result in serious functional deficit. When persistent deformity without ongoing inflammation is the dominant feature of the impairment, it should be evaluated under 1.02, or, if there has been surgical reconstruction, 1.03.

a. In 14.09A, the term <u>major joints</u> refers to the major peripheral joints, which are the hip, knee, shoulder, elbow, wrist-hand, and ankle-foot, as opposed to other peripheral joints (e.g., the joints of the hand or forefoot) or axial joints (i.e., the joints of the spine.) The wrist and hand are considered together as one major joint, as are the ankle and foot. Since only the ankle joint, which consists of the juncture of the bones of the lower leg (tibia and fibula) with the hindfoot (tarsal bones), but not the forefoot, is crucial to weight bearing, the ankle and foot are considered separately in evaluating weight bearing.

b. The terms *inability to ambulate effectively* and *inability to perform fine and gross movements effectively* in 14.09A and must have lasted, or be expected to last, for at least 12 months.

c. Inability to ambulate effectively is implicit in 14.09B. Even though individuals who demonstrate the findings of 14.09B will not ordinarily require bilateral upper limb assistance, the required ankylosis of the cervical or dorsolumbar spine will result in an extreme loss of the ability to see ahead, above, and to the side.

d. As in 14.02 through 14.06, **extra-articular features of an inflammatory arthritis may satisfy the criteria for a listing in an involved extra-articular body system.** Such impairments may be found to meet a criterion of 14.09C. Extra-articular impairments of lesser severity should be evaluated under 14.09D and 14.09E. **Commonly occurring extra-articular impairments include keratoconjunctivitis sicca, uveitis, iridocyclitis, pleuritis, pulmonary fibrosis or nodules, restrictive lung disease, pericarditis, myocarditis, cardiac arrhythmias, aortic valve insufficiency, coronary arteritis, Raynaud's phenomena, systemic vasculitis, amyloidosis of the kidney, chronic anemia, thrombocytopenia, hypersplenism with compromised immune competence (Felty's syndrome), peripheral neuropathy,** radiculopathy, spinal cord or cauda equina compression with sensory and motor loss, and heel enthesopathy with functionally limiting pain.

e. The fact that an individual is dependent on steroids, or any other drug, for the control of inflammatory arthritis is, in and of itself, insufficient to find disability. Advances in the treatment of inflammatory connective tissue disease and in the administration of steroids for its treatment have corrected some of the previously disabling consequences of continuous steroid use. Therefore, each case must be evaluated on its own merits, taking into consideration the severity of the underlying impairment and any adverse effects of treatment.

<u>**Systemic vasculitis (14.03)**</u> - This disease occurs acutely in association with adverse drug reactions, certain chronic infections and, occasionally, malignancies. More often it is idiopathic and chronic. There are several clinical patterns, including classical polyarteritis nodosa, aortic arch arteritis, giant cell arteritis, Wegener's granulomatosis, and vasculitis associated with other connective tissue disorders (e.g., rheumatoid arthritis, SLE, Sjogren's syndrome, cryoglobulinemia). Cutaneous vasculitis may or may

not be associated with systemic involvement and the patterns of vascular and ischemic involvement are highly variable. The diagnosis is confirmed by angiography or tissue biopsy when the disease is suspected clinically. Most patients who are stated to have this disease will have the results of the confirmatory angiogram or biopsy in their medical records.

Undifferentiated connective tissue disorder (14.06) - This listing includes syndromes with clinical and immunologic features of several connective tissue disorders, but that do not satisfy the criteria for any of the disorders described; for instance, the individual may have clinical features of systemic lupus erythematosus and systemic vasculitis, and the serologic findings of rheumatoid arthritis. It also includes overlap syndromes with clinical features of more than one established connective tissue disorder. For example, the individual may have features of both rheumatoid arthritis and scleroderma. The correct designation of this disorder is important for assessment of prognosis.

Disability Evaluation Under Social Security

Evidentiary Requirements: Medical Evidence under both the title II and title XVI programs is the cornerstone for the determination of disability. Each person who files a disability claim is responsible for providing medical evidence showing that he or she has an impairment(s) and how severe the impairment(s) is/are. However, SSA will help claimants get medical reports from their own medical sources when the claimants give SSA permission to do so. This medical evidence generally comes from sources who have treated or evaluated the claimant for his or her impairment(s).

Acceptable Medical Sources: These generally include licensed physicians (including licensed osteopaths), licensed or certified psychologists, and licensed optometrists (for measurement of visual acuity and visual fields). Social Security also requests copies of medical evidence from hospitals, clinics, or other health facilities where a claimant has been treated. All medical reports received are considered during the disability determination process.

Medical Evidence from Treating Sources: Currently, many disability claims are decided on the basis of medical evidence from treating sources. SSA regulations place special emphasis on evidence from treating sources because they are likely to be the medical professionals most able to provide a detailed long-term picture of the claimant's impairments, and may bring a unique perspective to the medical evidence that cannot be obtained from the medical findings alone, or from reports of individual examinations or brief hospitalizations. Timely, accurate, and adequate medical reports from treating sources accelerate the processing of the claim.

Other Evidence: Information from other sources may also help show the extent to which a person's impairment(s) affect(s) his or her ability to function. Other sources include public and private social welfare agencies, non-medical sources such as teachers, day care providers, social workers and employers, and other practitioners such as naturopaths, chiropractors, audiologists, and speech and language pathologists.

Medical Reports: Physicians, psychologists, and other health professionals are frequently asked by SSA to submit reports about an individual's impairment. Therefore, it is important to know what evidence SSA needs.

Medical reports should include:

* medical history
* clinical findings (such as the results of physical or mental status examinations)
* laboratory findings (such as blood pressure, x-rays)
* diagnosis
* treatment prescribed, with response and prognosis
* a statement providing an opinion about what the claimant can still do despite his or her impairment(s), based on the medical source's findings on the above factors. This statement should describe, but is not limited to, the individual's ability to perform work-related activities, such as sitting, standing, walking, lifting, carrying, handling objects, hearing, speaking, and traveling. In cases involving mental impairments, it should describe the individual's ability to understand, to carry out and remember instructions, and to respond appropriately to supervision, coworkers, and work pressures in a work setting. For a child, the statement should describe his or her functional limitations in learning, motor functioning, performing self-care activities, communicating, socializing, and completing tasks (and, if a child is a newborn or young infant from birth to age 1, responsiveness to stimuli).

Consultative Examinations: If the evidence provided by the claimant's own medical sources is inadequate to determine if he or she is disabled, additional medical information may be sought by re-contacting the treating source for additional information or clarification, or by arranging for a Consultative Examination (CE). The treating source is the preferred source for a CE if he or she is qualified, equipped, and willing to perform the examination for the authorized fee.

Evidence Relating to Symptoms: In developing evidence of the effects of symptoms, such as pain, shortness of breath, or fatigue, on a claimant's ability to function, SSA investigates all avenues presented that relate to the complaints. These include information provided by treating and other sources regarding:

* the claimant's daily activities
* the location, duration, frequency, and intensity of the pain or other symptom
* precipitating and aggravating factors
* the type, dosage, effectiveness, and side effects of any medication
* treatments, other than medications, for the relief of pain or other symptoms
* any measures the claimant uses or has used to relieve pain or other symptoms; and
* other factors concerning the claimant's functional limitations due to pain or other symptoms.

In assessing the claimant's pain or other symptoms, the decision-maker(s) must give full consideration to all of the above-mentioned factors. It is important that medical sources address these factors in the reports they provide.

Applying for disability benefits in the United Kingdom

*The following information is reprinted with permission from the Benefitsnow website at **www.benefitsnow.co.uk**. Additional information can be received by contacting The Benefitsnow Partnership, Silver Mist, Victoria Street, Ventnor, Isle of Wight, PO38 1ES **Telephone:** 07967 196690.*

What is DLA and Attendance Allowance?

DLA (Disability Living Allowance) is designed to help those people with severe disabilities to be better able to look after themselves. The two components (care and mobility) for disability living allowance are intended to cover all aspects of the ways which in which people may be affected by disability. Attendance Allowance is paid to people over the age of 65 who need help with personal care, or who need a lot of looking after. There is no mobility component for Attendance Allowance, and some have argued that this discriminates against older people.

What's good about DLA and Attendance Allowance?

Both are universal benefits- it doesn't matter whether you are rich or poor- you get paid according to your needs.

You don't have to obtain a doctor's report when you apply, although self-reporting does mean that some people understate their needs.

The care component is based on what you need, rather than on your medical condition.

You can spend your benefit on anything you want

What's wrong with DLA and Attendance Allowance?

Some of the terms used in the criteria are imprecise and can lead to confusion ("virtually unable to walk," "for the purpose of watching over you" etc).

Appealing against a decision can be a long and costly process.

Access to decent information about DLA is hard to locate- most of the published information is either simplistic, or overly dense and wordy.

The application pack for DLA is 44 pages long, ; some people are put off by this.

It still takes the DSS over two months to process an application.

The absence of a mobility component for Attendance Allowance discriminates against older people.

Some people feel that the medical assessment process is insufficiently independent.

How to Get an Application Pack

You need an application pack (ref DLA 1, or DLA 1 (Child) for children), for which you can telephone the Benefits Enquiry line on 0800 882200, or ask for one at your local DSS office (you can find this from the DSS site at **www.dss.gov.uk**). You can also get an Application Pack from your local Citizens Advice Bureau.

Filling out the forms

Try to be as accurate as possible.

Try to clearly explain the type of help that you need, and when you need it.

Anybody can help you to fill out the form. If you wish, a DSS advisor will fill out the form and send it to you to check and sign.

Give as much information as you can: particularly the medical name for your condition if you know it.

Write down everything that is wrong with you, not just the main problem.

When you are listing your medications, write down what strength or quantity it is and how many times a day you take it.

It is often helpful to put in the name of your hospital consultant if you have one: the adjudication officer might want to ask them about you to obtain a clearer picture of your needs.

Remember that the person who reads the form has not met you, so try to give a clear and detailed word-picture of your needs and difficulties.

It is very important to try to write something in every large white box that applies to you.

Don't assume that the adjudication officer knows about your condition, or its symptoms and effect. Give lots of description and detail, even about things that you find embarrassing or seem too trivial.

Mobility needs

It is much better for your case if you know exactly how far you can walk before you start experiencing "severe discomfort" or pain. Do your own walking test to measure the distance you can walk, and time yourself doing it. Note down your symptoms while walking, such as pain, fatigue or breathlessness. It is useful to say what you think could happen if you did go out alone in a place you didn't know, or to describe a previous incident where something dangerous could have happened.

Care Needs

The adjudication officer needs to know about how you cope during both the day and night. Again, it is very important to give as much detail as you can, and to write something in every box that applies to you.

You should describe your needs as fully as possible. Obviously, you stand much more chance of succeeding if you can show that you need help on most, or all, days of the week. Make sure you give lots of information and detail about the help you need, even if it is repetitive or embarrassing. Try to give an idea of what might happen if you didn't have that help, and include examples of past events if you can. On the form you should stress that you need the help even if you don't actually receive any. Explain that if you had a carer, they would always have to help you do things that you currently struggle to do yourself. For example, someone might help you have a bath twice a week. This does not mean you only need help to bathe twice a week. If you cannot have a bath on your own, it is reasonable to say you need help with this activity seven days a week.

You need to make it clear what you think might happen if you didn't have supervision or someone keeping an eye on you. Describe any past incidents that could have had serious consequences if you hadn't had help. Put down on the form what you fear might happen if you were left alone for long periods. If you have fits or falls describe what happens as vividly as you can, and how you cope afterwards. Falls are highly relevant. Describe how your carer or friend has helped you in the past after a fit or a fall.

Always describe in detail what happens to you during the night and how you have to be helped. For instance, needing to be helped to the toilet might involve being helped out of bed, helped to the toilet with your carer waiting outside the toilet while you use it, and then helping you back into bed and making sure you are comfortable. This can take quite a few minutes each time, so make sure the Adjudication Officer knows as much about your case as you do! If you need help with medication during the night, describe what might happen if you did not get it.

Read through the form and make sure you have described everything as fully and clearly as you can. Your claim will be dated from the date that you asked for the form.

How to get a decision changed:

There are three ways you can try to get a decision changed:

You can ask the DSS to revise their decision. You can ask for a revision for any reason at all.

You can ask the DSS to supersede their decision. Decisions are superseded if there has been a significant change in your circumstances since you first claimed, or if the DSS has made a mistake in deciding your claim.

You can appeal to an independent tribunal.

Time limits

You should ask for a revision within 4 weeks of receiving the DSS decision (6 weeks if you ask for a written explanation). There is no time limit on asking for a decision to be superseded. You should ask for an appeal within 4 weeks of receiving the original decision, or on receiving a decision on a revision or a supersession (6 weeks if you ask for a written explanation).

Complaints

If you are not satisfied with the service the DSS have given you, get leaflet GL22 (*“Tell us your comments and complaints”*) from your social security office. For your nearest social security office, look for the Benefits Agency display advert in the business numbers section of the phone book, or use the local office service on the DSS web site.

APPENDIX 4

Behçet's organizations

These addresses and phone numbers were correct as of April 2002. If you encounter any difficulties in contacting these groups, you may wish to check my master list at ***www.behcetsdisease.com/links.htm*** for updated information.

American Behçet's Disease Association (ABDA)
PO Box 15247
Chattanooga, TN 37415
www.behcets.com
Phone: 1-800-723-4238

Behçet's Syndrome Society (U.K.)
3 Church Close
Lambourn
HUNGERFORD
Berks RG17 8PU
UNITED KINGDOM
www.behcets.org.uk
Tel: 01488 71116
info@behcets-society.fsnet.co.uk

International Society for Behçet's Disease
(Physician and health care professionals group)
Contact Address:
President: Dr. Colin G. Barnes
Little Hoopem
Chagford TQ 13 8BZ
UNITED KINGDOM
www.behcet.ws
Tel: +44 1647 +432098
Fax: +44 1647 432097
 cgbarnes@btinternet.com

Behçet Israel Group (BIG)
www.behçet.org.il
Contact Tal Kinnersley for more information:
big@behçet.org.il
This site includes extensive information in English on alternative and complementary treatments for Behçet's.

Appendix 4

French Behçet's Association
(Associatio de B7)
24, rue Amiral Duchaffault
85600 MONTAIGU
FRANCE
Tel : 02 28 15 04 73
www.behcet.asso.fr
E-mail: contact@behcet.asso.fr

Germany
Selbsthilfegruppe "Leben mit Behçet"
Adeltraud Müller
Wilhelmsthaler Strasse 2
34125 Kassel
GERMANY
Phone: +49 (0)561 875751

Italian Behçet's Association
www.behcet.it
For information, contact
Massimo Nicolardi at info@behcet.it

Japan
Hokkaido Behçet's Association
Ms. Sachiko Hirata
Nishi 10-chome
Minami 4-jo
Chuo-ku, Sapporo
Hokkaido 064-8506
JAPAN
Phone: +81 (0)561 875751
ssappo@yahoo.co.jp

Osaka Behçet's Association
www.geocities.co.jp/HeartLand-Gaien/4572

Korean Behcet Support Association
www.behcet.co.kr
International liaison: liaison@behcet.co.kr

Turkish Association of Behçet's Patients
Çetin Ezber (Secretary)
IU Cerrahpasa Tip Fakultesi
Ic Hastaliklari Anabilim Dali
Romatoloji Bilim Dali
34303 Cerrahpasa
Istanbul
TURKEY
 Phone:+90 212 520 18 97

INDEX

About the Author:

Joanne Zeis is a member of the American Behçet's Disease Association, and the International Society for Behçet's Disease. She holds a B.S. in Psychology from Tufts University, with additional classes through the Continuing Education Department of Harvard Medical School and the Mind/Body Medical Institute. Her previous works include *You Are Not Alone: 15 People with Behçet's*, *Basic Information on Behçet's Disease*, and *Behçet's Disease: Medical Research Studies*. She resides in Massachusetts with her husband and two children, and has been living with Behçet's disease since 1979.